EAT

TO PREVENT
AND CONTROL
DISEASE

How Superfoods Can Help You Live Disease Free

LA FONCEUR

Eb
emerald books

Eb
emerald books

Dear reader,

The aim of **Eat to Prevent and Control Disease** is to help reduce your dependence on medicines by providing you with in-depth knowledge of common chronic diseases as well as the best food options that prevent and control diseases naturally.

Eat healthily, live happily!

Master of Pharmacy, RPh

and Research scientist

.

CONTENTS

INTRODUCTION

Nowadays, diabetes, high blood pressure, and arthritis have become quite common. One in every family has one of these diseases. People have started considering these diseases as part of life, which is not good. The lifestyle we are leading today - high intake of processed foods, frequent eating out, smoking, and alcohol, there is a 70% chance that you will have either high blood sugar levels or high blood pressure or both by your 50s.

A disease state in the body means your immune system is constantly busy fighting the disease, soon your immune system loses its effectiveness and becomes weak. If another disease strikes, your immune system is unable to fight, this can have life-threatening consequences. It is very important to start as early as in your 20s to take care of your health. Make your body strong enough to fight any disease naturally.

More diseases mean more medicines. Being from a pharmacy background, I can assure you that dependence on medicines is not good. Medicines prescribed in disease have side effects. To reduce side effects, you are often prescribed with another set of medicines that treat the side effects of your primary medications, but they also have side effects, for which again some other medications are required, so basically, this cycle continues. But there is a solution! You can include foods in your diet that have the same effect as your medications. By regular intake of these foods, you can heal your body and increase your immunity to fight disease naturally.

The objective should be to prevent disease, and preparation starts in your 20s. What you eat in your 20s affects your 50s. To prevent a disease, you must have a thorough knowledge of the disease, such as why it happens? How does it affect your body? What exactly does happen in your body in the event of a disease? What are other health problems that can be caused by a particular disease?

In *Eat to Prevent and Control Disease*, all these topics will be discussed in detail. You will learn about foods that boost your immunity, superfoods that can protect you from diseases, foods that reduce inflammation in your body, and food combinations that you should eat for maximum health benefits.

You will also learn everything about the three most common chronic diseases- diabetes, high blood pressure, and arthritis. To prevent these diseases, which foods and lifestyle options should you avoid, and which ones should you adopt? What should be your strategy to prevent and control these diseases. What are the foods that mimic your medication's mechanism of action and can help lower your blood pressure and sugar levels? What are the key points that you can follow to prevent arthritis and get rid of it?

You will also discover some healthy and tasty recipes that have all the healthy ingredients and still very tasty. These recipes will strengthen your immunity as well as satisfy your taste bud. Get ready for a healthy tomorrow!

UNIT 1

EAT TO PREVENT DISEASE

1

ROLE OF FOOD THERAPY IN PREVENTING AND CONTROLLING DISEASE

Role of food therapy in preventing and controlling disease

If you have your blood sugar levels checked for the first time, and your report says that your blood sugar is high, your doctor will not first prescribe you the medicines. Instead, your doctor will give you a three-month time so that you can control your sugar with diet and lifestyle modifications. If the blood sugar is still not controlled, then only you will be prescribed with medicines to control high sugar levels.

You know why? Because medicines treat disease, but they can cause strong side effects. The stronger the drug, the stronger will be its side effects. It doesn't mean you should stop taking medicines without informing your doctor. Never stop your medication without consulting your doctor because some medicines have withdrawal effects, which can even worsen your disease condition if you stop taking them suddenly.

So, what is the solution? The solution lies in good management. You can prevent or manage the disease only when you have comprehensive knowledge about that disease. Everything is on your hand, and you are the commander of your life and your disease condition. With the correct nutrition and healthy lifestyle, you require fewer medicines, shorter therapy duration, and minimum side effects.

When it comes to disease management, there are lots of misconceptions associated with it. Let's first clear these misconceptions:

#1 Misconception

I am young, and I don't have any disease, I have plenty of time to live without worrying. I will worry about diseases when I will hit my 50. Till then, my motto is *You Only Live Once*.

Actually, you only die once but live every day, so make your every day disease-free. The age of 20 to 40 is your key to make your 50+ years healthy and happy. The way you treat your body between these years, its effect is seen in your old age. These are your sowing years, eat as many healthy foods as you can during these years, and reap the benefits in your 50+ years. Strictly avoid smoking, alcohol, and other drugs that deteriorate your health internally. The harm never visible during your 20s and 30s, but it has life-threatening consequences soon after you hit your 50s or nowadays even in your 40s. Eat junk foods but only to satisfy your taste bud, definitely not to fill your tummy.

#2 Misconception

I am a very health-conscious person, and I believe nature has all the solutions. Although I have been diagnosed with a disease, but I believe I don't need medication. I can heal myself naturally with healthy food and a good lifestyle.

If you have been diagnosed with a disease means the harm has unknowingly already been done. Keep in mind medicines are not the enemy, just they are not a natural food. Sole dependence on medicines is not good; at the same time, completely abandoning medicines when your body needs them is also not right. No doubt, healthy foods, and healthy lifestyle choices can heal you much faster, but you definitely need medication to treat a disease. With healthy foods, you can heal yourself faster, and your body recovers more quickly, so you need a shorter course of therapy that simply means lesser side effects.

#3 Misconception

Last time when I had these symptoms, my doctor prescribed these medicines. Now again, I feel the same problem, I should take the same medicines as the doctor had prescribed me last time.

Avoid self-medication. In a condition of reoccurrence of any disease, medicines may be the same, but with different doses. Don't be a doctor yourself. Self-medication may result in an overdose, which can lead to toxicity and other life-threatening consequences. Seek advice from your doctor every time you are not feeling well and ask him/her directly if it is safe to take the same medication again when the symptoms occur. Always ask your doctor about what should be the diet in managing your disease? Ask your pharmacist if there is any food that you should avoid while taking the prescribed medicine.

#4 Misconception

I was on medication, and my condition has improved. Although my doctor had prescribed me a 3-month course of medicines, I was feeling fine, so after two months, I stopped taking the medicines.

This is never advised. Maybe with your healthy diet and lifestyle, you have recovered faster than others, but you should never leave your medication course in between without consulting your doctor. Even if your symptoms are relieved with initial medications, you need the full course to treat the disease completely. Otherwise, it will reoccur, and as it has not been treated in the initial stage, it will reoccur with more severeness. Abruptly discontinuing some medicines produce withdrawal effects in the body and worsen the disease condition. Instead of quitting your medicines, you should inform your doctor about your improvement. Your doctor will gradually reduce the dose of the same medication and complete the course sooner than before, or he will advise you to complete the full course depending upon your disease type and your condition.

#5 Misconception

I am taking medicine for my illness, and medicine is doing its job. It will cure me, I don't have to worry too much about nutrition and all.

Food and lifestyle play a huge role in managing any disease. If your diet is not healthy and your lifestyle is also not good, then your condition may worsen despite regular medication. Foods that boost immunity prepare your body to fight the disease and heal your body. A healthy lifestyle removes the burden from your body; hence your body can completely focus on treating the disease.

#6 Misconception

Some diseases like diabetes, high blood pressure, arthritis, etc. come naturally with age. You cannot escape from these diseases. Every other person I know has one of these diseases, so this is pretty normal at my age.

It may be common but indeed not normal. This is the biggest myth that some diseases naturally come with age. With age, our body becomes a little weaker, but most of these diseases are the result of our poor diet and poor lifestyle. It's time to stop letting these diseases become part of your life and build your body with healthy foods and a healthy lifestyle in such a way that these diseases never even touch you, and if you already have these diseases, then they can be controlled.

DISEASE MANAGEMENT

What is a disease?

A disease is a condition of disturbances in the normal structure or function of your body. When something goes wrong with the normal function of your body, your body gives signals in the form of signs and symptoms that something is going wrong inside the body. This is where your responsibility begins. With proper medication, healthy foods, and healthy lifestyle, you can prevent and treat disease.

Disease is mainly managed with medications and foods and lifestyle modifications. Let's understand the role of each.

ROLE OF MEDICATIONS

Prescribed medications play a vital role in the treatment. Generally, medicines work in three ways:

1. To reduce symptoms like pain, nausea, and fever.

2. To treat the disease.

3. To reduce or treat the side effects arising due to the use of medicines in curing the disease. Such as antacids are usually prescribed with high dose medications as these medications can cause acidity in the body.

It is important to take the medicines at the same time every day. Medicines take their time (onset time) to show their effect on the body. Taking medicines at the same time every day ensures that its active ingredient will be available in the body uniformly throughout the treatment.

ROLE OF LIFESTYLE CHOICES

Poor lifestyle choices give a burden to your body. In simple terms, these are the inducer of many diseases. Unhealthy lifestyle choices weaken your body, lower your immunity, and make you susceptible to many diseases.

Example of unhealthy lifestyle choices:

Stress

Smoking

Alcohol

Unhygienic habits

Inadequate sleep

When it comes to poor lifestyle choices, you may have found plenty of discussions about smoking, alcohol, and inadequate sleep, but we often take other poor lifestyle choices such as stress and unhygienic habits lightly.

Stress is a key contributor to many diseases. When you are under stress, your body releases the stress hormone cortisol, which causes your heart to pump faster and raises your blood pressure. After the stressful time has passed, your body releases lower amounts of cortisol. Your heart and blood pressure return to normal. But if you are under constant stress, the consistently high levels of cortisol in your body can cause many health problems. Take out at least 2 hours for yourself every day, do nothing during this time, just relax. Just two stress-free hours in a day gives your body enough time to normalize all its functions and systems.

Unhygienic habits such as not washing your hands before eating and after using the washroom, and touching an open wound allow germs to enter the body. As a result, your immune system keeps busy fighting these germs and with time immune system weakens. When your immune system becomes weak, it can't protect you from major and serious diseases. So, don't stress out your immune system. Already there is so much pollution in the environment with which your immune system fights daily, so do not give it more burden. Maintain good hygiene and keep your immune system healthy. Whenever you come from outside, first wash your hands with soap water. This habit will protect you from many diseases. Also, 5-Second rule is a big myth. Even a brief exposure of the floor can contaminate your food with E. coli, salmonella, and other bacteria in under five seconds.

What should be your focus points to prevent disease?

If you keep your immune system and digestive system healthy, you greatly lower your risk of diseases.

Avoid Immune weakening lifestyle choices

- Stress
- Smoking
- Drinking Alcohol
- Consuming narcotics such as Cannabis

Adapt the immune-boosting lifestyle choices

- 7-8 hours of sleep
- Washing your hands frequently
- Expose yourself to early morning sunlight
- Yoga
- Taking a walk after lunch and dinner

Avoid immune weakening foods

- Trans fats
- Processed foods
- Canned foods
- Refined carbohydrates

- Foods high in sugar

Add immune-boosting foods in your diet

- Foods rich in vitamin C

- Foods high in zinc

- Foods that have anti-inflammatory effects

ROLE OF FOODS

Foods play a massive role in every stage of disease management. These roles include:

1. To prevent the disease.

2. To shorten the therapy period.

3. To control the disease.

4. To prevent the reoccurrence of the disease.

Body is nature's product, and your body loves natural things like food. Plant-based healthy foods can prevent various diseases and autoimmune disorders and help build your body strong enough to fight off any disease. Plant-based healthy foods heal your body, reduce your dependency on medicines, and add disease-free years to your life.

Why food therapy is the best therapy?

Medicines work on the disturbance that has been arisen in your body dues to disease, while foods work on the root cause and strengthen your body to fight with the disease naturally. Moreover, foods have no side effects. A simple rule is to include vegetables and fruits of every color in your diet; it will protect you from countless diseases.

We are so concerned about avoiding unhealthy foods that it has become quite stressful now. The more you try to run away from them, the more you crave. If you do not eat unhealthy foods, but your diet lacks essential nutrients, then there is no health benefit of avoiding unhealthy foods. To stay healthy, incorporating healthy foods into your diet is more important than just avoiding unhealthy foods. It is time to focus on what you should eat, not what you should not eat. Do not modify your diet for weight loss; instead, balance your diet for a healthy and disease-free life.

2

10 SUPERFOODS YOU MUST EAT EVERY DAY TO LIVE DISEASE-FREE

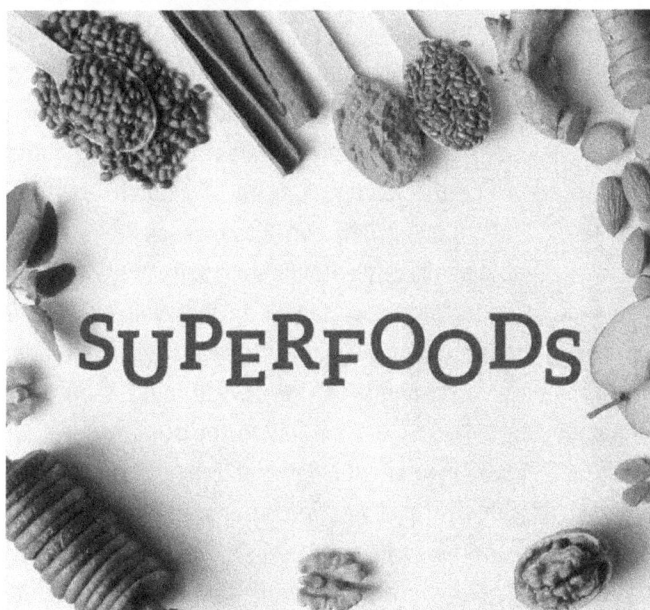

10 superfoods you must eat every day to live disease-free

Foods can protect you from many diseases and can improve your disease condition. Superfoods are foods that are highly dense in nutrients. A food is considered as a superfood when it not only can protect or treat a single disease, but its regular consumption can protect you against many diseases at a time. Eating just superfoods and avoiding other foods doesn't guaranty you a disease-free life. But eating superfoods every day definitely reduces the risk of developing the disease manifold. This is because superfoods contain active chemical compounds that are antioxidant and anti-inflammatory, and inhibit oxidative stress by killing free radicals and reduce inflammation in the body. Oxidative stress and inflammation are the leading causes of cancer, arthritis, diabetes, and many such chronic diseases. You can prevent these diseases by eating superfoods every day. Do not look at superfoods as medicines that you only need until your condition improves. See them as lifelong friends; They are here to do good for you, so you must keep their company throughout life. I am listing top superfoods that you must include in your everyday diet. But to stay disease-free, you should also avoid eating processed foods, canned foods, fried items, salt, and other well-known health deteriorators. Here are superfoods that have medicinal properties and can reduce your dependency on medicines. Let's meet our lifelong food friends:

TURMERIC

Turmeric deserves to be at the top of the superfoods list. Turmeric has scientifically proven health benefits. The credit goes to curcumin, the active compound of turmeric. Curcumin gives the bright yellow color to turmeric and has many medicinal properties. It is a potent anti-inflammatory, antioxidant, antibacterial, antiviral, and antifungal agent. These properties play an important role in keeping your body strong enough from inside to prevent most of the disease.

Inflammation is good for the body as it helps heal an injury or fights infection, but our today's food and lifestyle cause inflammation in the body at a dangerous level. Chronic inflammation is one of the reasons for almost every disease, including arthritis, heart disease, Alzheimer's disease, depression, cancer, and other degenerative conditions. Curcumin has potent anti-inflammatory property which protects you from many diseases. Lower levels of Brain-Derived Neurotrophic

Factor (BDNF) is associated with Alzheimer's and depression. Turmeric boosts the levels of BDNF and very effective in preventing and treating depression and Alzheimer's disease.

Turmeric helps prevent and control a variety of cancer types, including prostate, breast, colorectal, and pancreatic cancers. It helps stop the growth of tumor cells.

Due to its antibacterial and antiviral property, curcumin might help fight off infection and a variety of viruses, including herpes and viral flu. So, next time when you get a viral fever, add one tablespoon of turmeric powder in milk, boil for two minutes, and drink it before bed. It will heal you faster.

Turmeric protects cells from the damage caused by free radicals. Unhealthy foods like foods high in saturated fats, sugar as well as poor lifestyle choices such as drinking alcohol contribute to free radicals, which is associated with tissue damage. Free radicals can cause damage to cells of DNA, proteins, and cell membranes, by pairing with their electrons through the oxidation process. These are responsible for aging and other health complications. Turmeric has a high content of polyphenols, flavonoids, tannins, and ascorbic acid; these all are the natural antioxidants and help protect cells from the damage caused by free radicals.

How to consume turmeric?

Eat fresh turmeric in the winter season. Grate it and add in your morning tea. In other seasons, use turmeric powder in cooking and have hot turmeric milk at night before bed. Turmeric is warm in nature, so don't overeat it in summer, you may get mouth ulcer.

Who should avoid turmeric?

No one. It can consume by anyone. Eat black pepper with turmeric; it increases curcumin absorption in the body. However, if you are taking blood-thinning medicines like warfarin, you should limit your turmeric consumption because turmeric purifies the blood and thins the blood.

How much turmeric should I eat in a day?

You should aim to get 500mg-1000mg of curcumin in a day, which is equivalent to one tablespoon of freshly ground turmeric or one tablespoon of turmeric powder. Avoid supplements rather than go for fresh or powdered turmeric.

FENUGREEK LEAVES AND SEEDS

Fenugreek leaves and seeds have a wide range of nutrients that provide numerous health benefits. They are packed with iron, vitamins, biotin, choline, flavonoids, and fibers. The high antioxidant flavonoid content in fenugreek seeds can reduce pain and inflammation and improve arthritis conditions. Fenugreek leaves and seeds are high in soluble fiber, which helps lower blood sugar and decreases cholesterol levels. The fiber in fenugreek slows down the digestion and absorption of carbohydrates and is very effective in controlling diabetes. High blood cholesterol levels increase your risk of heart diseases. The soluble fiber in fenugreek gets attached to cholesterol particles and takes them out from the body, thus decreasing the cholesterol levels in the body and reduces blood pressure. This reduces the risk of developing heart complications and improves heart health.

Also, fenugreek seeds are effective in the treatment of hair loss, male impotence, and other types of sexual dysfunction.

How much fenugreek should I consume in a day?
One teaspoon of fenugreek seeds in a day for six months to see the result. Aim to eat fresh fenugreek leaves every day or every alternate day in the winter season.

What is the best way to consume fenugreek?

Soak one teaspoon of fenugreek seeds in a glass of water overnight. Next morning, chew the fenugreek seeds and swallow them with a full glass of water (in which seeds were soaked). Make fresh fenugreek leaves salad or sauté them in mustard oil, add garlic to enhance the taste.

Who should avoid fenugreek?

If you are on medication of diabetes or hypertension, don't start taking fenugreek in high amount without consulting your doctor and pharmacist. Fenugreek may perform similar functions as your diabetes and BP medications. So taking both may lower blood glucose and blood pressure below the safe range. Because of that, the dose of your medicines might need to be changed.

FLAX SEEDS

Flax seeds are probably the healthiest among all the seeds. They have got the reputation of superfood because they are packed with cancer-fighting polyphenols lignans, alpha-linolenic acid (ALA), and fibers. Flax seeds contain approximately 100 times more lignans than any other plant foods, which helps in protecting against breast cancer, colon cancer, and prostate cancer. They are one of the best sources of an omega-3 fatty called acid alpha-linolenic acid (ALA). Due to their high omega-3 content, they help reduce the risk of heart disease, stroke, and diabetes through their anti-inflammatory action. Omega-3 fatty acid alpha-linolenic acids, along with lignans, block the release of pro-inflammatory agents and reduce inflammation in the body. The anti-cancer property of flax seeds is due to their lignans content; they suppress the growth, size, and spread of cancer cells by blocking enzymes that are involved in hormone metabolism.

How much flax seeds should I eat in a day?

One tablespoon (10g-15g) of flax seeds in a day.

What is the best way to eat flax seeds?

Dry roast and grind them. Add the ground flax seeds in chapati and tortilla dough.

Who should avoid flax seeds?

There are no side effects reported till date, so it is safe to eat flax seeds for all. Always remember moderation is the key. Consuming too much flax seeds with too little water can worsen constipation and may lead to an intestinal blockage, so take flax seeds with plenty of water to prevent this from happening.

SWEET POTATOES

Sweet potatoes are one of the best sources of beta carotene that converts into vitamin A in the body and promote eye health as well as boost immunity. Beta carotene functions as a potent antioxidant that reduces cell damage and helps prevent the free radical damage that is associated with cancer. The higher fiber content of sweet potatoes prevents constipation and promotes a well-functioning digestive tract. The presence of anthocyanin pigments in sweet potatoes, particularly in purple-fleshed sweet potatoes, helps in preventing and reducing chronic inflammation in the body.

Sweet potatoes are rich in both magnesium and potassium, both of which are essential in lowering blood pressure and reduce the risk of cardiovascular diseases.

Higher fiber and magnesium content of sweet potatoes may decrease diabetes risk. Moreover, sweet potatoes help to regulate the blood sugar levels, especially in people with diabetes; its high insoluble fibers content promotes insulin sensitivity. Unlike other starchy foods, sweet potatoes have a low glycemic index. They release sugar into the bloodstream slowly and steady, which aids in controlling the blood sugar levels of individuals.

How many sweet potatoes should I eat in a day?

One medium sweet potato in a day is enough to meet your daily recommended vitamin A intake.

What is the best way to cook sweet potatoes?

To get the most nutrition from your sweet potatoes, don't peel them, simply wash, and scrub well before cooking. They can be boiled, steamed, and baked. Steamed or boiled sweet potatoes have more healthy benefits than baked sweet potatoes because baking releases the sugar inside the sweet potato, which may increase blood glucose levels.

Who should avoid eating sweet potatoes?

People who have existing kidney stones or are at high risk of developing them or those who are on dialysis should avoid sweet potatoes. It is because sweet potatoes are high in potassium, and when you have kidney disease, your kidneys cannot remove extra potassium, and too much potassium can stay in your blood.

COW'S MILK

The reason why you should drink milk every day is because cow's milk is a complete food means it contains every nutrient that you need in a day for a healthy body. Cow's milk is packed with protein, calcium, potassium, vitamin A, B vitamins, and phosphorous. When you feel hungry, have a glass of cow's milk, it's enough to give you energy for the next 2 -3 hours.

Let's see why milk is so good for your health:

Amino acids are compounds that combine to make proteins. Your body needs nine essential amino acids through food to maintain normal functioning. Not all protein sources are considered as a high-quality complete protein because not all protein-rich foods contain all nine essential amino acids. Milk is a rich source of protein, mainly casein (80%) and whey (20%). Both are considered as complete protein because both contain all nine essential amino acids that are required for your body to maintain good health.

Milk is an excellent source of calcium, which is necessary to build healthy bones and teeth and to maintain bone mass. The presence of vitamin D in milk increases the absorption of calcium in the body. Calcium with vitamin D can protect you from osteoporosis.

Magnesium and potassium in milk support proper kidney and heart function and can help you prevent hypertension and heart diseases.

Milk is a complete package; you can get all essential nutrients in a single, convenient source. If you are thinking of switching to vegan, keep in mind that it is hard to have all milk's nutrients in a single vegan food source. Most of the vegan sources are fortified means extra nutrients are manually added to them, and these nutrients are not naturally present in them, so basically, these are not natural sources. Also, when you switch to vegan, you need supplements to reach daily vitamins and minerals need of the body, which is an effective way but again, not the natural way. Anything which is not natural is not advised to be dependent on for a long time.

Milk products that you should add in your diet:

Cow's milk (best for health), low-fat yogurt, buttermilk, cottage cheese, and cow's milk's ghee.

Milk products that you should avoid:

Heavy cream, processed cheese, and whole-fat dairy products.

How much milk and milk products should I consume in a day?

250 ml cow's milk + 2-3 milk products (yogurt, cottage cheese).

Who should avoid milk?

If you are lactose intolerant, you should avoid milk. Another alternative is lactose-free cow's milk, which contains all the nutrients of milk, but it's free from lactose. Lactose-free cow's milk is made by adding the enzyme lactase to cow's milk, which breaks down the lactose into glucose and makes it lactose-free and can easily be digested by lactose-intolerant people.

Limit your dairy consumption in the wet season. Consuming too much dairy can aggravate gastric problems, cause nausea, diarrhea, and stomach pains, even though if you are not lactose intolerant. So, moderation is the key.

If you have a cough, limit your milk and milk product consumption. Avoid taking milk at night. Milk doesn't increase the production of phlegm, but it can make your existing phlegm thicker and may irritate your throat and aggravate a cough.

RAW GARLIC

Garlic is an adaptogen which means it stabilizes and maintains a steady internal environment in the body, in response to environmental changes. It ensures the optimal functioning of the body, including the regulation of body temperature, blood sugar, blood pressure, pH balance, and functioning of the immune system. This is the reason why initially garlic had used for medicinal purposes only. Most of the potent medicinal properties of garlic are due to the allicin, a sulfur compound that gives pungent smell to the garlic. The thing with allicin is that it only releases when you crush or cut the garlic. Allicin is very unstable, which means you need to use it immediately after you cut garlic. The allicin in raw crushed garlic is destroyed by heat. So, for health benefits, eat fresh raw garlic.

Also, garlic protects against bowel and stomach cancers. It is scientifically proven that the sulfur components of garlic alter the biological behavior of tumors, tumor microenvironments, and precancerous cells. Garlic decreases cancer risk, particularly cancers of the gastrointestinal tract.

Garlic is known to contain natural antioxidants that can eliminate low-density lipoprotein (LDL) cholesterol from the body and help protect against heart disease by thinning the blood and improve blood circulation. Garlic reduces both systolic and diastolic blood pressure by increasing the nitric oxide production in the body, which helps smooth muscles to relax and widen the blood vessels.

The antibacterial and antifungal properties of garlic help fight infections and boost the function of the immune system. So basically, this vegetable (yes, it's vegetable, not an herb or spice) can actually protect you from many diseases. It's time to add RAW garlic in your diet!

How should I take garlic?

Eat one clove of freshly crushed raw garlic every morning on an empty stomach. Don't eat more than one clove of fresh raw garlic at a time. Don't keep garlic in the mouth for too long; it may cause burn. Eat plenty of garlic (raw and cooked) in winter, add them in soup or spring roll. Limit garlic consumption in the summer season, too much of garlic in summer, may result in acne and ulcer due to its heat-producing nature.

When should I avoid garlic?

If you have ulcers, colitis, acid reflux, or heartburn problem, limit your garlic consumption.

How much garlic is enough for health benefits?

One clove of raw garlic (crushed) on an empty stomach every day is enough. If you experience heat, ulcer or acid reflux, then instead of daily, eat it twice or thrice a week.

SPROUTS

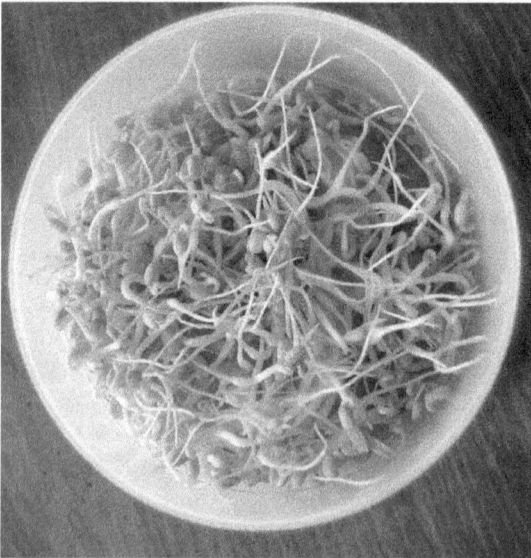

Sprouts are affordable, safe, and easily grown nutrient-dense superfood. Sprouting can increase nutrition up to 100 times than raw legumes and vegetables.

For those who have difficulty digesting certain foods, sprouting is a better option for them. The reason is sprouting increases the proteolytic enzymes content of the food that break down starches into simpler carbohydrates, proteins into amino acids, and fats into fatty acids. So, your digestive system need not break them, which makes these nutrients more bioavailable and easily digestible.

Why is sprouting beneficial for you? Because sprouting increases the nutrition value of legumes and vegetables, it removes enzyme inhibitors and unlocked healthy compounds. The increased bioavailability of high levels of vitamins, minerals, amino acids, essential fatty acids, and antioxidants increases the alkalinity of your body. Raising pH (to an alkaline state) increases the ability of your immune system to prevent disease.

Grow sprouts at your home to reduce your exposure to pesticides, food additives, and other chemicals. There are so many different sprouts varieties you can try, including mung bean, black chickpeas, lentils, wheat sprouts, alfalfa, radish seeds, and broccoli.

How many sprouts should I eat in a day?

Eat a bowl of different varieties of sprouts in a day. You don't need to eat the same sprouts every day, keep them rotating, eat every sprout on alternate or every three days, but try to have a bowl of sprouts every day.

What is the best way to eat sprouts?

Eating them raw will keep all the nutrients locked. To make them tangy, add finely chopped cucumbers, onions, tomatoes, fresh-squeezed lemon juice, black salt, and black pepper.

Who should avoid eating sprouts?

In case you are going for store-bought sprouts (which I would not recommend at all), don't eat them raw. Cook them thoroughly until steaming hot throughout to reduce the risk of food poisoning from Salmonella, Listeria, or E. coli. Store-bought sprouts can be contaminated anywhere along the journey from farm to table. People with weakened immune systems should not eat any variety of raw or lightly-cooked sprouts; it may result in food poisoning.

SPINACH

Spinach is called a superfood because of its anti-inflammatory and antioxidant properties. It is packed with iron, vitamin k, protein, calcium, magnesium, and potassium that protect your body from a wide range of diseases. Spinach is a significant source of vitamin K, which is an important factor in wound healing and bone health. Spinach is rich in carotenoids that are beneficial antioxidants that boost your immune system. It contains three different types of carotenoids: beta carotenoid, lutein, and zeaxanthin.

Beta carotenoid converts into vitamin A in the body and has a vital role in maintaining healthy vision, healthy immune system, and healthy reproduction system. Lutein and zeaxanthin function as a light filter, protecting your eye tissues from UV rays of sunlight.

The high levels of potassium in spinach, along with folate, relaxes the blood vessels and lower your blood pressure. Spinach also helps the body make nitric oxide, a natural vasodilator which further lowers blood pressure.

Often people who have type 2 diabetes have low levels of magnesium. Spinach is very low in calories and has a low glycemic index. Additionally, it is rich in magnesium, which helps to lower blood sugar and can even protect you from type 2 diabetes.

What is the best way of eating spinach?

The more you cook spinach, the more it will lose its nutrients. Either sauté the spinach or blanch the spinach, but don't blanch for more than 1 minute. Add lemon juice while blanching, it will increase the absorption of nutrients in your body, and you will get the full health benefit.

Who should not eat spinach?

Limit your spinach consumption if you have kidneys stone or if you are at a high risk of developing kidney stones because spinach is high in both calcium and oxalates that can cause kidney stones.

If you are taking blood-thinning medication, do let your doctor and pharmacist know about your spinach consumption. Spinach is high in vitamin K that promotes blood clotting and can decrease the effectiveness of your blood-thinning medication such as warfarin.

DRY FRUITS

You must have heard this 1000 times that you should eat nuts every day! But do you follow it? If not, then it's time to start eating nuts every day! Eating dry fruits every day helps promote overall well-being and ensures a healthy, disease-free long life. Nuts contain heart-friendly monounsaturated and polyunsaturated fats, and antioxidants like flavonoids and vitamin E. Research suggests that high consumption of nuts, including peanuts, is associated with two to three times reduced risk of breast cancer.

Dry fruits are high in fiber and magnesium, which help to stabilize blood sugar and insulin levels. Dry fruits lower the risk of developing type 2 diabetes.

Dates are loaded with iron and potassium and yet contain little sodium, which helps maintain normal blood pressure and keeps the risk of a stroke in check.

Dried figs are a good source of calcium. Figs keep bodily systems like the endocrine, immune, respiratory, digestive, and reproductive system in check.

Almonds are an excellent source of vitamin E, protein, and monounsaturated fats. They promote weight loss by reducing hunger and keeping you full for a longer period. The healthy fats and antioxidants of almond lower blood pressure and cholesterol levels and also lower the blood sugar levels.

Walnut kernels don't just look like a brain, but they actually contain brain-boosting polyphenolic compounds like omega-3 fatty acids. Polyphenols are considered critical brain food and prevent cognitive disorders.

Cashew nuts are rich in zinc, which boost immunity and prevent male pattern baldness and prostate enlargement by blocking the creation of Dihydrotestosterone (DHT).

How many dry fruits should I eat in a day?

Eat a handful of different dry fruits every day, including almond, walnut, cashew nuts, pistachio, dates, raisins, and figs. Frequency matters, so it is important to eat them every day even if the quantity is less than a handful.

What is the best way to eat dry fruits?

Nuts contain phytic acid that reduces the nutrition value of nuts by lowering absorption, so the best way to remove phytic acid is soaking. Soak a handful of dry fruits in water overnight and eat them the next morning.

Who should avoid eating dry fruits?

You should eat plenty of dry fruits in winter but limit your dry fruits consumption in the summer season. Nuts produce heat in the body, while it is beneficial in winter to keep you warm; in summer, it can give you acne, ulcer, and acidity.

BASIL LEAVES

Holy basil or tulsi is a superfood because it is an immunomodulator and adaptogen. It lowers blood sugar levels, cholesterol, and triglycerides.

Stress increases your risk of developing or worsens conditions like hypertension, diabetes, heart disease, Alzheimer's disease, depression, obesity, and gastrointestinal problems. Adaptogen with anti-inflammatory properties of basil helps you to reduce stress, anxiety, depression, and very effective in preventing and treating cognitive disorders, including amnesia and dementia. The neuroprotective, anti-stress, and anti-inflammatory activities of basil enhance memory and improve brain function. For this reason, basil considers as a natural memory tonic.

Regular consumption of basil leaves can prevent viral infections. Research confirms that holy basil has an immunomodulatory effect; it increases the percentage of T-helper cells as well as NK-cells (Natural killer cells), which are the components of the adaptive immune system and innate immune system, respectively. These cells help eliminate pathogens by preventing their growth and help fight viral infections.

Research shows basil leaves are as effective in lowering blood glucose as antidiabetic drugs. Basil leaves have hypoglycemic properties, which lower blood sugar levels and improve insulin sensitivity. If you have prediabetes or type 2 diabetes, the essential oil of basil helps cut down cholesterol and triglyceride levels, which is a persistent risk factor for type 2 diabetes.

How much basil should I consume in a day?

Start your day by chewing two to three fresh basil leaves.

What is the best way to eat basil leaves?

Add 2-3 fresh basil leaves in your morning green tea. You don't need much expertise in growing basil at your home.

Who should avoid eating basil leaves?

Limit your basil consumption if you are taking medications like acetaminophen or paracetamol (pain reliever). If you are consuming plenty of basil leaves and taking paracetamol, they both work together and tend to affect the functioning of your liver.

CONCLUSION

Now that you know the foods that can naturally protect you from diseases, should you just opt for their dietary supplement? Not at all. Supplements are never recommended in place of natural foods. This is because the supplements contain ingredients that have strong biological effects in the body. Their dose may interfere with medications you may already be taking, which can sometimes have harmful consequences. Taking too much of some supplements can have life-threatening consequences. You should include various natural foods in your diet, not human-made foods, so supplements are a big no in replacing superfoods.

3

10 POWER FOODS TO BOOST YOUR IMMUNITY

10 power foods to boost your immunity

Keeping your immune system healthy, directly means protecting yourself from many diseases. In winter, cold and flu are quite common but have you ever thought why few people get flu while others not. The reason is their immunity. Some people have a naturally strong immune system, while others have weak. No matter whether your immunity is naturally strong or weak, you can definitely boost your immunity with some power foods. This will not only make your winter flu-free, but it will also protect you from many diseases.

When it comes to immunity, the four major nutrients that need to be taken into consideration are as follow:

Vitamin C is the most crucial nutrient for boosting your immunity. Vitamin C supports various cellular functions of the immune system, thus contributes to immune defense.

Vitamin A promotes as well as regulates the immune system. Therefore, it enhances the immune function and provides an enhanced defense against multiple infectious diseases.

Vitamin E is a potent antioxidant and can modulate immune functions. Studies suggest vitamin E improves the decreased immunity in aged people.

Omega-3 fatty acids are anti-inflammatory means they prevent inflammation or swelling in the body.

Zinc is an essential mineral that is crucial for the normal development and function of cells mediating immunity.

These four nutrients are crucial for maintaining and boosting immunity. A deficiency in any of these nutrients may weaken your immune system. Eating foods rich in zinc, omega-3, vitamin A, C, and E, help you build a stronger immune system. Let's see which power foods contain an abundance of these crucial nutrients.

Below are the 10 power foods to boost your immunity, so, start adding them in your diet for a disease-free, healthier life:

1. Citrus fruits

If you think of immunity, the first name that comes in your mind is vitamin C! and why not? Vitamin C is actually the best nutrient when it comes to immunity. It protects against immune system deficiencies, skin wrinkling, cardiovascular disease, eye disease, etc. Vitamin C increases the production of white blood cells, which are an essential part of the immune system. These are the key to fight infections by killing bacteria and viruses that invade the body. Citrus fruits such as lemon, tangerine, orange, and grapefruit are high in Vitamin C.

Citrus fruits are a natural antioxidant that boosts the immune system. These have antiviral and antibacterial properties that prevent infections, bacterial growth, and relieves nausea.

Squeeze one medium lemon in one glass of warm water (250 ml) and drink it every morning. You need vitamin C daily for continued health, so make a habit of taking lemon water instead of plain water every morning.

2. Turmeric

This bright yellow spice is a natural immunomodulator that boosts your immunity. Curcumin, the active compound of turmeric has many scientifically-proven health benefits. Curcumin is a potent antioxidant and has anti-inflammatory effects. Turmeric not only boost your immunity but also very effective in treating both rheumatoid arthritis and osteoarthritis. Add one tablespoon of turmeric powder in hot milk (250 ml) and drink it every night just before bed and see the magic yourself.

3. Garlic

Garlic is an adaptogen, which means it helps the body to adapt varied environmental and psychological stresses and supports all the major systems, such as the nervous system, immune system, and hormonal system. It regulates blood sugar; if they are too high, it will lower it and vice-versa.

Garlic contains active compound allicin that improves the immune cells' ability to fight off the flu and reduces the risk of infection. Garlic also has anti-inflammatory, antibacterial, and antiviral properties that help in inhibiting the growth of some bacteria and fight against viral infections.

Taking one clove of crushed garlic on an empty stomach every day not only boosts your immunity but also normalizes all major systems in your body. If your body is already acidic or warm in nature, limit the consumption to 3 times a week.

4. Ginger

The bioactive substance gingerol in the ginger root has anti-inflammatory and anti-fungal properties. It helps in lowering the risk of infections and relieving a sore throat. It also helps fight viruses such as rhinoviruses, human respiratory syncytial virus (HRSV), which cause colds, and many respiratory infections. Ginger is a strong antioxidant, it naturally boosts your immunity. Drinking ginger tea every morning in the winter season keeps you warm and saves you from cold and flu.

5. Flax seeds

Flax seeds are rich in Omega-3 fats that help protect your body against bacteria and viruses, improving your immunity. Flax seeds contain the highest concentrations of dietary lignans that help protect against cancer by blocking the growth and spread of tumor cells. These are also a great source of iron that ensures your immune system gets required oxygen to fight infection. The omega-3 fatty acids of flax seeds fight inflammation in the body and prevent inflammatory diseases such as rheumatoid arthritis, psoriasis, and lupus.

6. Red and green bell peppers

If you think orange or lemon is the richest source of vitamin C, then here is the surprise, bell peppers contain twice as much vitamin C as any citrus fruit. They are also a rich source of beta carotene, which converts into vitamin A in your body. The high content of both vitamin C and vitamin A in bell peppers enhance your immune function and provide enhanced defense against multiple infectious diseases. Vitamin A is an anti-inflammation vitamin that helps in treating and preventing arthritis and contact dermatitis. Eat cooked bell peppers because cooking increases vitamin C content in bell peppers.

7. Cashews

Cashews are a great source of zinc and copper. Zinc plays an important role in the production of immune cells and antioxidant enzymes that help fight disease and infection. Cashews have antioxidant effects that help your body fight off oxidative damage. Cashews speed up the healing of wounds as they are rich in vitamin K. Vitamin E of cashews help decrease inflammation in your body. Pregnant women must eat cashews as they help with the growth and development of the baby.

8. Papaya

Papaya has antioxidant and immunostimulant effects that reduce oxidative stress and improve immune functions. Papayas also contain potent antioxidants known as carotenoids — particularly lycopene. Carotenoids are converted into vitamin A in the body and help regulate the immune system. Papaya is also a great source of vitamin B, C, and K and known as an excellent immunity booster. It slows down the aging process and helps your skin look more youthful and supple. One medium-sized papaya can fulfill your daily requirement of vitamin A.

9. Yogurt

It is said that the healthier your gut is, the better will be your immunity. Yogurt is the best probiotic. Yogurt contains lactobacillus, a probiotic, or good bacteria that help keep your gut healthy, also gives your immune system a boost. Yogurt is also high with vitamins and protein. Due to the immunostimulatory effects of yogurt, it helps fight against diseases such as infection, GI disorders, cancer, and asthma. It is actually very beneficial for older people.

Go for plain yogurt, not the flavored ones, and eat it with your lunch.

10. Green tea

The list is incomplete without the mention of green tea. The higher concentration of polyphenols and flavonoids, the two powerful antioxidants, make green tea a gem for boosting your immunity. These antioxidants kill the free radicals in the body and increase your longevity.

Free radicals are the by-products of the process where cells use oxygen to generate energy in the body. At low or moderate levels, free radicals are harmless, but at high concentrations, they cause oxidative stress, a deleterious process that can damage all cell structures. Oxidative stress plays a crucial role in the development of arthritis, autoimmune disorders, cancer, aging, cardiovascular and neurodegenerative diseases.

The powerful antioxidants in green tea kill these free radicals and help in fighting illnesses, like common cold, arthritis, aging, and cancer. Start drinking green tea if you have not started yet!

CONCLUSION

These foods definitely boost your immunity, but to keep your immune system healthy, it is also important to have a healthy lifestyle that includes getting sufficient sleep, doing yoga, taking a morning walk, and managing your stress. Definitely, there are dietary supplements available in the market to boost your immunity, but their effects are limited. One good thing about going natural is, it comes with all benefits with no side effects. Most of the immune booster foods also enhance your skin and hair health, so it's a win-win situation.

4

10 NUTRIENT COMBINATIONS YOU SHOULD EAT FOR MAXIMUM HEALTH BENEFITS

10 nutrient combinations you should eat for maximum health benefits

Nutrients need to adequately absorbed into your body to provide health benefits. Some nutrients are eliminated faster from your body without being absorbed, and you don't get their health benefits. Various factors affect the absorption of nutrients. Foods require a favorable environment inside your body and the presence of certain vitamins and minerals to get absorbed. If foods don't get absorbed in your body, you don't get the health benefits. Fortunately, you can enhance the absorption of food by pairing it with other food that can provide an environment required for their absorption and prevent their metabolism, making the nutrient more available in the blood to get absorbed. Eating these foods together ensures that you get maximum health benefits.

Below are 10 nutrient combinations that you should eat for maximum health benefits.

1. Vitamin C + Iron

Iron is an essential nutrient required for blood production. Hemoglobin of red blood cells comprises about 70 percent of iron. Hemoglobin transfers oxygen through your blood from the lungs to the tissues. Deficiency in iron may cause iron-deficiency anemia that can lead to heart problems. You may become deficient in iron if you are eating too little iron-rich foods, or the iron is not getting absorbed properly in the body. When you eat vitamin C with iron, it increases the stability and solubility of iron by binding with them. Once iron becomes more soluble, it allows the body to more readily absorb the iron through the mucus membranes of the intestine.

Food combinations that you should eat for better iron absorption:

1. Lemon juice + Spinach

Add lemon juice when blanching the spinach, it will retain the dark green color of spinach as well as increase the iron absorption.

2. Lemon juice + Sprouts

3. Tomatoes + Lentils

4. Orange + Oatmeal

5. Tomatoes + Beetroot

2. Vitamin D + Calcium

Calcium and vitamin D both are very important for your bone health. Not only your bones but your heart, muscles, and nerves also need calcium to function properly. You must have noticed that the prescribed calcium tablets always come in a combination of vitamin D. There is a solid reason behind it. Vitamin D is the fat-soluble nutrient that increases the absorption of calcium in the intestine. Calcium, along with vitamin D, not only can protect you against osteoporosis and bone disease. This combination can even protect against diabetes, high blood pressure, and cancer.

Food combinations that you should eat for better calcium absorption:

1. Expose your skin to sunlight for 10 to 15 mins in the morning after that drink a glass of milk.

2. Mushrooms + Soybeans

3. Yogurt + Nuts

4. Mushrooms + Dark leafy greens

5. Sour cream + Broccoli

3. Turmeric + Black pepper

Turmeric has health benefits due to its active compound curcumin. The problem with curcumin is its poor absorption in the body. Additionally, curcumin is rapidly metabolized in the body that leads to its rapid elimination from the body. As a result, you could be missing out on its health benefits. By combining turmeric and black pepper, you can increase curcumin bioavailability. Black pepper has active ingredient piperine that protects curcumin from the digestive enzymes. It slows down the breakdown of curcumin. As a result, curcumin remains in the bloodstream for a longer period. It, therefore, boosts the absorption of curcumin by multiple times, making it more readily available to be used by the body.

4. Zinc + Vitamin A

Vitamin A is not only crucial for protecting against night blindness, but it also promotes healthy growth and development and has a very critical role in enhancing immune function. Absorption of vitamin A is hugely affected by zinc availability in the body. Zinc plays a vital role in the absorption, transporting, and utilization of vitamin A in the body. When your body is deficient in zinc, it affects the movability of vitamin A from the liver to body tissues. Zinc also regulates the conversion of retinol (vitamin A) to retinal that requires the action of a zinc-dependent enzyme. So, if you eat vitamin A-rich foods together with zinc-rich foods, you will get the maximum health benefits of vitamin A.

Food combinations that you should eat for better vitamin A absorption:

1. Cashew nuts + Carrot cake

2. Legumes + Spinach

3. Dry fruits + Mango milkshake

4. Swiss cheese + Sweet potato

5. Oats + Papaya

5. Green tea + Lemon

Green tea is loaded with catechins which are the polyphenols that have potent antioxidative, anti-inflammatory, and antibacterial activity. Catechins improve blood pressure, blood sugar levels, prevent cell damage and very effective in preventing cancer. The catechins of green tea are relatively unstable in the intestine. Vitamin C rich foods such as citrus fruits increase the amount of catechins available for the body to absorb. Vitamin C interacts with catechins to prevent their degradation in the intestines. As a result, more catechins are available to absorbed in the body. So, make sure to add lemon juice in your green tea because when you add lemon in your green tea, it increases catechins absorption by more than five times.

6. Phytic acid + Water

Plant-based foods such as whole grains, legumes, and nuts contain phytic acid that binds with minerals such as iron, zinc, calcium, and manganese and prevents their absorption in the body. When phytic acid binds with these minerals, it forms phytates, and our bodies do not have any enzymes that can break down phytates to release these minerals. So, you don't get the full health benefits of these minerals. Fortunately, the simple solution to this problem is soaking! Soaking in water allows the phytic acids to leach onto the water. You should soak phytic acid-containing foods in water overnight (or for at least 3-4 hours). It will increase the bioavailability of the minerals and decrease gastrointestinal distress.

Foods that you should soak for better absorption:

1. Nuts (Almond, peanuts, walnuts, and others)

2. Legumes (kidney beans, chickpeas, and peas)

3. Rice

4. Wheat bran

5. Sesame

7. Tomato + Olive oil

Lycopene is the main carotenoid in tomatoes. The antioxidant lycopene of tomatoes is responsible for reducing the risk of heart disease and certain types of cancer. Lycopene is a fat-soluble compound, which means it is better absorbed in the presence of healthy fat. Eating tomatoes cooked in olive oil greatly increase the absorption of lycopene and protect your cells against free radicals, which play a role in aging, heart disease, cancer, and other diseases.

8. Folate + Vitamin B12

Folate (Folic acid or vitamin B9), when taken alone, can mask the symptoms of vitamin B12 deficiency. The problem is that without symptoms, you will not know that you are deficient in vitamin B12. This can delay the diagnosis, and there could be a risk of developing nerve damage. Because of this reason, these vitamins are often taken together. Moreover, folate works closely with vitamin B12 to make red blood cells and to help iron function properly in the body. Folate and vitamin B12 together (along with vitamin B6) help lower homocysteine levels. Study shows high levels of homocysteine (an amino acid) are associated with the development of coronary artery disease, leading to heart attacks and strokes. If you eat folate and vitamin B12 rich foods together, you will never get deficient in folate or vitamin B12, and you will never get depressed because these two vitamins, when eaten together, enhance the immune function and mood.

Folate and vitamin B12 food combinations that you should eat for maximum health benefits:

1. Yogurt + Banana

2. Shiitake mushrooms + Dark leafy greens

3. Milk + Nuts

4. Yogurt + cooked Okra (Ladyfinger)

5. Whey + Lentils

Whey is the by-product of cottage cheese-making. It is the liquid remaining after milk has been curdled and strained. Cook lentils in whey instead of plain water.

9. Rice + Beans (complete protein)

The human body needs nine amino acids, which are essential means you need to get them through food. A complete protein means a food source of protein that contains an adequate amount of each of the nine essential amino acids. Not all protein sources are a complete protein, especially vegetarian protein sources. That doesn't mean being a vegetarian, you will miss out on amino acids. When you eat correct food combinations, you can get all the essential amino acids. The best example is rice and beans. Together, rice and beans form a complete protein because when eaten together, they provide all nine essential amino acids necessary in the human diet.

Beans are rich in lysine but missing an amino acid known as methionine. Rice has high levels of methionine but doesn't have enough amino acid lysine. When rice and beans (such as kidney beans and chickpeas) are consumed together, each provides the amino acid that the other lacks, making it a high-quality protein. Here are some more high protein food combinations.

Food combinations that you should eat to get complete protein:

1. Kidney beans + Rice

2. Green peas + Lentils

3. Corn + Mixed beans

4. Red lentils + Brown rice

5. Cabbage + Wheat

10. Vitamins A, D, E and K + Healthy fats

Vitamin A, D, E, and K all are fat-soluble vitamins. These fat-soluble vitamins require the availability of fat to absorb properly in the body. Your body can't absorb them effectively without eating some fat at the same time. Some examples of foods containing fat-soluble vitamins are mango, red bell peppers, sweet potato, and most of the colored vegetables (vitamin A), milk and milk products (Vitamin D), almonds, peanuts, sunflower seeds (vitamin E) and leafy greens like spinach, kale, cauliflower (Vitamin K).

Food combinations that you should eat for better absorption of fat-soluble vitamins:

1. Almond milkshake

2. Nuts roasted in cow's ghee

3. Spinach + Mustard oil

4. Mango + Avocado

5. Nuts + Flaxseeds

CONCLUSION

It is not very hard to eat the food combinations mentioned above. Some of the above food combinations you might already be eating, some combinations might be new to you. It's time to do some experiments with your taste bud. If you come up with a new dish while combining these nutrients, do let me know. I would love to try it too.

UNIT 2

DISEASE: PREVENTION AND CONTROL

Diabetes

Hypertension

Arthritis

1
<u>DIABETES</u>

1.1

EVERYTHING YOU NEED TO KNOW ABOUT DIABETES

Everything you need to know about diabetes

Diabetes is probably the most common chronic disease; 1 in 11 of the world's adult population is living with diabetes. It's like a slow poison. It slowly affects the other part of your body and a major cause of kidney failure, blindness, and heart attacks. The worrying part is people don't take diabetes seriously. The younger generation is not well educated about it, and affected people are highly dependent upon medicines, giving less effort on diet and exercise front. Diabetes doesn't come with age, but it comes with a bad lifestyle and diet deficient in healthy nutrients. If you have type 2 diabetes, you don't need to live with it; diabetes is reversible. Early diagnosis, a healthy diet, physical activity, and medications can help you reverse diabetes. If you have diabetes for a long time and you are on high dose medications, your aim should not be just to avoid sugary foods. You should aim to eat foods that mimic the action of your anti-diabetic drugs and exhibit similar effects in the body and also have no side effects. Regular screening of diabetes complications can help you prevent and treat complications before they become severe.

Here are some dangerous facts about diabetes that no one talks about:

- According to the International diabetes federation, diabetes caused 4.2 million deaths in 2019.

- 374 million people are at increased risk of developing type 2 diabetes, according to IDF.

- According to WHO, diabetes is a major cause of kidney failure, heart attacks, stroke, and blindness.

- Diabetes was the seventh leading cause of death in 2016, according to WHO.

Don't just accept diabetes as a new normal; it may be common but not normal. Let's prevent and control diabetes through natural ways. But for that, first, you need to have thorough knowledge about every aspect of diabetes so that with a little help from health professionals (who can guide you at every step where you will have confusion), you can prevent and control diabetes without medicines.

What is diabetes?

Diabetes is a chronic disease, it occurs either when the body does not produce insulin or does not effectively use the insulin it produces. Insulin is a hormone that helps the body use sugar for energy. Hyperglycemia is the medical term for high blood sugar (glucose) levels. It is a common effect of uncontrolled diabetes. Over time, hyperglycemia leads to severe damage to many of the body's systems, especially the nerves and blood vessels.

Types of diabetes:

TYPES OF DIABETES

©La Fonceur

DIABETES INSIPIDUS

People with diabetes insipidus have normal blood glucose levels. The only similarity between diabetes mellitus and diabetes insipidus is excessive urination. Diabetes insipidus occurs when kidneys cannot balance fluid in the body. It happens due to some damage in the pituitary gland, which releases the anti-diuretic hormone (ADH), also known as vasopressin. ADH or vasopressin enables the kidneys to retain water in the body. In the absence of vasopressin, kidneys excrete too much water. This causes frequent and excessive urination and can lead to dehydration.

DIABETES MELLITUS

Diabetes mellitus, or simply diabetes, is a disorder that is characterized by abnormally high blood sugar (glucose) levels because the body does not have enough insulin to meet its needs. It is caused either because the body doesn't produce enough insulin or because the body is ineffective in using insulin. In diabetes, urination and thirst are increased and damages the nerves and tiny blood vessels that cause health complications, especially in the kidneys and eyes.

What happens in your body in diabetes?

When you eat food containing carbohydrates, your body breaks them down into sugar (glucose) and send that to your bloodstream. The rise in glucose triggers the pancreas to release insulin into the bloodstream. Insulin signals muscle, liver, and fat cells to take in glucose from the blood. These cells then convert glucose into energy or store it for later use. In diabetes mellitus, your body doesn't use insulin as it should, which results in too much glucose in your blood.

Type 1 diabetes

(Insulin-dependent diabetes)

Type 1 diabetes is an autoimmune condition in which the pancreas cannot produce insulin. Typically, the immune system protects your body against the attack of bacteria and viruses by fighting against them. An autoimmune condition is a condition in which your immune system mistakenly attacks your body's cells. In type 1 diabetes, the immune system destroys the beta cells of the pancreas that produce insulin, making the pancreas unable to produce insulin.

Insulin is a hormone that regulates the blood sugar levels in your body. In the absence of insulin, your body can't use or store glucose for energy. The glucose stays in your blood, and your blood sugar or blood glucose levels become too high (hyperglycemia). Persistent high glucose levels result in diabetes and can lead to complications affecting your kidneys, nerves, eyes, and heart. A person who has type 1 diabetes requires daily insulin injections to control blood glucose.

The condition usually appears in children and young people, so it used to be called juvenile diabetes.

Type 2 diabetes

(Insulin-independent diabetes)

Type 2 diabetes is the most common form of diabetes that primarily occurs due to obesity and lack of exercise. It is characterized by high blood sugar (hyperglycemia) and insulin resistance.

Insulin resistance means your pancreas is releasing insulin as it should, but the cells in your muscles, fat, and liver start resisting the signal given by insulin to take glucose out of the bloodstream for making energy. This results in too much glucose in your blood, known as prediabetes.

In a person with prediabetes, the pancreas works increasingly hard to release enough insulin to overcome the body's resistance and to keep blood sugar levels down. Over time, the pancreas' ability to release insulin begins to decrease, which leads to the development of type 2 diabetes.

Reason for Insulin resistance

The driving forces behind insulin resistance are excess body weight, too much fat in the abdominal area, and a sedentary lifestyle, while genetics and aging also play a role in developing insulin resistance.

GESTATIONAL DIABETES

Gestational diabetes is a condition in which your blood glucose levels become high during pregnancy. Body goes through different changes during pregnancy, such as weight gain and changes in hormones, which affects the body's cells' ability to respond to insulin effectively. Most of the time pancreas can produce enough insulin to overcome insulin resistance, but some pregnant women cannot produce enough insulin and develop gestational diabetes. Mostly, gestational diabetes goes away soon after delivery. Women who develop gestational diabetes during pregnancy are at higher risk of developing type 2 diabetes later in life.

Here is everything about diabetes mellitus that you need to know to prevent and control it:

SYMPTOMS OF DIABETES:

Excessive urination (polyuria): To get rid of excess glucose, kidney makes more urine than usual. Daily urine output can be more than 3 liters a day compared to the normal urine output about 1 to 2 liters.

Excessive thirst (polydipsia): Too much glucose forces kidneys to work overtime. Kidneys pull water from tissues to make more urine to help pass the extra glucose from your body, which makes you dehydrated. This usually makes you feel very thirsty.

Fatigue: Because the body's cells do not get enough glucose to make energy.

Weight loss (in Type I diabetes): Because of dehydration caused by excessive urination and loss of calories from the sugar that couldn't be used as energy.

Constant hunger: Because the body can't convert the food you eat into energy.

Blurred vision: High blood sugar causes body water to be pulled into the lens inside the eye, causing it to swell.

WHY IS DIABETES DANGEROUS?

Uncontrolled diabetes can lead to potential health complications, including:

Retinopathy (Eyes damage): High blood sugar levels can weaken and damage the small blood vessels of the retina, which can cause visual disturbance and can even lead to blindness.

Neuropathy (Nerve damage): Constant high blood sugar can damage nerves that typically results in numbness, weakness, tingling, and burning or pain, usually in the hands and feet (diabetic foot).

Nephropathy (kidney damage): Over time, diabetes can damage the small blood vessels in the kidneys, which can lead to kidney failure, and the person may require dialysis or a kidney transplant.

Ketoacidosis (mostly in Type 1 diabetes): When there isn't enough insulin in the body to convert glucose into energy, your body starts breaking down fat for energy. This process produces a build-up of acidic substances called ketones to dangerous levels in the body, eventually leading to ketoacidosis.

Heart disease: Over time, the high blood sugar levels can damage the blood vessels that maintain the heart function, causing them to become stiff and hard. A high-fat diet can cause a build-up of fats and cholesterol on the inside of these blood vessels, which can restrict blood flow. This condition is known as atherosclerosis. Atherosclerosis conditions can reduce blood flow to the heart muscles (which causes angina) and brain (which causes stroke) or can damage the heart muscle, which can result in a heart attack.

DIABETES: PREVENTION AND CONTROL

Diabetes condition can be effectively managed by

Diet

Medication

Exercise

Before going further, let's clear some terms associated with diabetes:

Glycemic index

You must have heard about low glycemic foods and high glycemic foods, but what is exactly the glycemic index?

The Glycemic index helps you differentiate between good carbohydrates and bad carbohydrates for diabetes. Not all carbohydrates are the same. Type of carbohydrates like complex carbohydrates takes longer to break down into glucose and slowly absorbed and metabolized that cause a slower rise in blood sugar. This type of carbohydrates doesn't give you a sudden spike of sugar levels and considered as good carbohydrates. These are categorized as low-glycemic foods; they help maintain good glucose control. Foods that have the glycemic value 55 or less are good for diabetes—for example, whole grains and beans.

Simple carbohydrates such as sugar and highly processed and refined carbohydrates such as pastries and cakes are considered as high glycemic foods. They speedily break down into glucose and quickly absorbed, causing a rapid rise in blood sugar. Repeated spikes in blood sugar lead to an increased risk for type 2 diabetes.

Hypoglycemia

Hypoglycemia condition is often caused by diabetes treatment. Hypoglycemia is the opposite of hyperglycemia. It is a condition in which your blood sugar levels are lower than normal. Certain diabetes medicines or too much insulin may cause your blood sugar levels to drop too low. It is a reversible condition and can be treated by consuming high-sugar foods such as fruit juice or honey. If you are on diabetes medication, you should pay attention to hypoglycemia symptoms, which include confusion, shakiness, and dizziness. If left untreated, hypoglycemia can get worse and can even cause seizures, coma, and death. Always keep glucose tablets with you in case you experience hypoglycemia.

ROLE OF MEDICATIONS IN DIABETES

How do diabetes medicines work?

Your most common and first choice of drug in diabetes (metformin) doesn't stimulate insulin secretion by beta cells in the pancreas; instead, it enhances the ability of your tissues to take glucose out of the bloodstream and convert it into energy, especially in muscles. Additionally, it lowers the production of glucose by the liver. It is a drug of choice because it doesn't cause weight gain and hypoglycemia. The common side effect of metformin is diarrhea. Don't just stop taking your medicine because of diarrhea; instead, eat yogurt, beans, an apple, or a banana (not more than one banana in a day) to prevent diarrhea. Make sure to drink plenty of water to prevent dehydration caused by diarrhea.

Another class of drugs (sulfonylureas), reduces high blood sugar by increasing insulin secretion by beta cells in the pancreas. Additionally, it increases cells' sensitivity to insulin, which increases the efficiency of the body's cells to take out glucose from the bloodstream. It also increases the availability of insulin in blood by reducing the degradation of insulin in the liver. The side effects of this class of drugs are weight gain and hypoglycemia. It is very important to keep an eye on your hypoglycemia symptoms, which include shakiness, sweating, dizziness, confusion, irritability, and loss of consciousness. Severe hypoglycemia can potentially lead to coma. Take glucose tablets (total 15g or ask your doctor for exact amount) or foods high in glucose like one tablespoon of honey or sugar or 3-4 raisins to treat hypoglycemia immediately. Ask your doctor to adjust the dose of your medicines if you experience hypoglycemia.

ROLE OF EXERCISE IN DIABETES

Obesity and diabetes connection

Obesity is a common reason for type 2 diabetes. Just by losing weight, you can prevent the onset of diabetes. If you are in the prediabetes stage, you can even reverse diabetes by losing weight, and by including hypoglycemic and weight-loss-friendly foods in your diet.

Excess fat may contribute to insulin resistance. It is because when your fat cells that store extra fat become too large, they stop storing fat. Additional fat starts storing in muscles, liver, and pancreas, making these organs resistant to insulin, and they stop responding to the signal given by insulin to take glucose. Moreover, fat cells decrease the secretion of adiponectin, a protein hormone that helps in the breakdown of fat. In simple terms, adiponectin is your fat-burning hormone. High adiponectin levels can protect you against insulin resistance, diabetes, and heart disease. The more you lose weight, the higher your adiponectin levels.

How can weight loss prevent the onset of diabetes?

In type 2 diabetes, insulin production decreases over a sustained period, and the process is rather slow in comparison to type 1 diabetes. It is possible that a strict diet and exercise regime, leading to weight loss, and may delay or even prevent the onset of diabetes. The key is to diagnose the diabetes condition before beta cells function deteriorates.

After the age of 40, you should get your sugar levels tested every year for early diagnosis of high blood sugar levels. If you are overweight, losing weight is your first and most crucial step. It will not only save you from diabetes but can protect you against many diseases. You don't need to lose weight in a short time. Start eating diabetes-friendly foods and start with moderate exercise, soon your body will get habitual of your new diet and exercise regime. It should not be your short-term goal but a new lifestyle.

Ideal weight target to prevent insulin resistance

Body mass index: 25 kg/m^2

Waist circumference: Less than 100 cm

ROLE OF DIET IN DIABETES

A healthy diet plays an important role in preventing and managing diabetes. Preventing diabetes isn't just about avoiding foods that can spike your blood sugar levels, it's also about choosing the right foods that naturally prevent diabetes. In diabetes, moderation and frequency are the keys, you can still eat your favorite foods, but you might need to eat them less often or eat smaller portions.

To prevent and control diabetes:

- Avoid sugary foods that directly raise your blood sugar levels.

- Avoid refined carbohydrates that quickly break down into glucose sugar and raise your blood sugar levels.

- Avoid foods that increase your risk of insulin resistance.

- Avoid foods that increase cholesterol in the body.

- Avoid lifestyle choices that increase the risk of developing diabetes.

- Avoid foods that increase your risk of developing diabetes complications.

Now that you know what type of foods you need to avoid, let's see in the next chapter, which are the top 10 foods and lifestyle choices that you should avoid to prevent and control diabetes.

1.2

10 FOODS THAT INCREASE YOUR DIABETES RISK

10 foods that increase your diabetes risk

Below are the 10 foods that can increase your diabetes risk:

1. Saturated fats

Saturated fats increase the risk of developing type 2 diabetes more than unsaturated fats. Foods that are high in saturated fats, such as butter, cheese, cream, and processed foods like cakes and biscuits can cause high levels of LDL-cholesterol, which increases the risk of cardiovascular diseases in people with diabetes. LDL-cholesterol transports from the liver to the cells, and fat build-up inside muscle cells lowers the insulin response to glucose and increases blood sugar levels, increasing the risk of developing diabetes. Foods like butter, coconut oil, palm oil, and cheese have high amounts of saturated fat.

2. Starchy foods

Starchy foods such as white rice, boiled potatoes, and pasta are high in glycemic index. These foods are quickly digested and absorbed, causing a rapid rise in blood sugar levels. The best way to reduce their effect is to replace them with healthier alternatives. These healthy alternatives contain fiber that is low in the glycemic index. You can replace white rice with brown rice, boiled white potatoes with sweet potatoes, and white pasta with whole wheat pasta or durum wheat pasta. Even though these healthy alternatives provide fiber, you should eat them in moderation.

3. Packaged fruit juices

Packaged fruit juices are high in fructose and low in fiber. It gives a sudden spike in blood sugar and is less nutritious than freshly squeezed juices. Unfortunately, even the healthiest packaged fruit juice in the market can increase insulin resistance and increase your risk of developing diabetes. In fact, not only packaged fruit juices, even fresh fruit juices are not healthy in comparison to fresh fruits. Most of the fibers, vitamins, and anti-oxidants are removed while filtering. So, it is best to eat whole fresh fruit instead of fruit juice.

4. Hydrogenated oils

Hydrogenated oils are mainly present in packaged food items such as peanut butter, french fries, margarine, ready-to-use dough, and readymade baked foods. Hydrogenated oils are nothing but healthy vegetable oils that are converted into unhealthier form by the food industry. Vegetable oils are liquids at room temperature, food manufacturers chemically alter the structure of vegetable oils and turn them into solid or spreadable form by adding hydrogen in them. As a result, trans fats are formed. Trans fats increase insulin resistance by affecting cell membrane functions and increase your risk of developing type 2 diabetes. They are a major contributor to heart disease because they are highly inflammatory and can increase your LDL-cholesterol (bad) while lowering your HDL-cholesterol (good).

5. Tobacco use

Tobacco use may fluctuate your glucose levels by altering the way your body uses glucose. Tobacco contains an addictive chemical called nicotine that increases insulin resistance, which can lead to type 2 diabetes. Tobacco stimulates the secretion of a steroid hormone called cortisol, which increases the production of glucose by the liver and makes fat and muscle cells resistant to the action of insulin. The more you smoke, the higher your risk of developing diabetes. Smokers have almost double the risk of developing diabetes compared with people who don't smoke.

6. Alcohol

Excess alcohol intake increases your risk of developing type 2 diabetes. Alcohol contains a lot of calories, which can make you obese. Obesity increases insulin resistance, which can lead to diabetes or can worsen your diabetes condition. Another disadvantage of drinking alcohol is that it produces a synergic effect and causes hypoglycemia by interacting with some of your prescribed anti-diabetic medicines such as sulfonylureas. Typically, the liver releases stored glucose when blood sugar levels drop, to maintain normal blood glucose, and to prevent hypoglycemia. But when you drink alcohol, it interferes with the way liver works and reduces the liver's ability to recover the dropped blood glucose levels. It results in hypoglycemia.

7. Soda

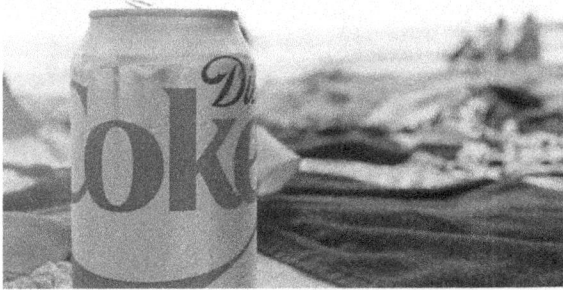

Soda and sugar-sweetened energy drinks can increase your diabetes risk, and if you already have diabetes, you must totally avoid them. The high sugar content of these drinks causes rapid spikes in blood sugar levels. These sugary drinks contain lots of calories, which can make you obese. The excess body weight makes your muscles, liver, and fat cells resistant to the insulin's signals of grabbing glucose out of the bloodstream. The high sugar levels in your blood make your pancreas to release more and more insulin to overcome the body's resistance and to maintain the blood sugar levels normal. Over time, this affects the pancreas's ability to make sufficient insulin, and your blood sugar begins to rise, and you develop diabetes.

8. Full fat dairy

Full-fat milk and milk products can increase the levels of cholesterol in the blood and lead to a higher risk of cardiovascular diseases. High-fat content can also lead to insulin resistance. Avoid eating full-fat milk, butter, full-fat yogurt, full-fat ice cream, and cheese. Even skimmed milk contains carbohydrates and can affect your blood sugar levels, but you should not completely avoid milk because it contains nutrients, which are a must for your body to function properly. It is better to remove other high calories and sugary food sources from your diet than milk.

9. Salt

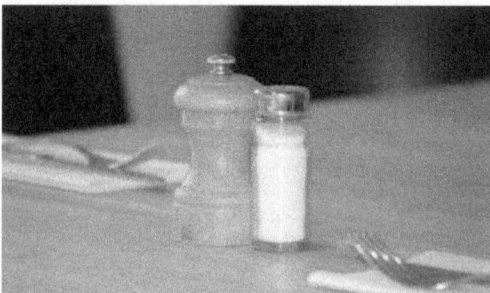

It is crucial to maintain normal blood pressure in diabetes. Salt does not directly affect blood glucose levels, but you should limit your salt consumption for managing diabetes efficiently. Too much salt can raise your blood pressure. High blood pressure with diabetes increases your risk of cardiovascular diseases. You should maintain your blood pressure less than 130/80 mm Hg. You must limit your table salt consumption to 5g or one teaspoon per day to prevent and control diabetes.

10. Certain drugs

Certain drugs such as corticosteroids and pain-relieving non-steroidal anti-inflammatory drugs (NSAIDs) are contradicted in diabetes. Oral Corticosteroids can increase blood glucose levels and cause insulin resistance by reducing the sensitivity of the cells toward insulin. Corticosteroids can worsen diabetes conditions; this is why people with diabetes, as well as individuals with pre-diabetes, should avoid them.

People with diabetes who are receiving sulfonylureas drugs should avoid taking a high dose of pain-relieving non-steroidal anti-inflammatory drugs (NSAIDs) such as ibuprofen. One of the side effects of sulfonylureas is hypoglycemia means it lowers the blood sugar levels than the normal range. NSAIDs affect the ion channel functions of beta cells that secrete insulin. When you take NSAIDs together with sulphonylureas, it induces hypoglycemia.

CONCLUSION

These were the foods and lifestyle choices that you must avoid or at least limit the consumption to prevent diabetes, but as I said before, just avoiding harmful foods is not enough in managing diabetes. You must eat the right nutrition; in fact, eating foods that naturally prevent and even treat your diabetes is more important than just avoiding harmful foods. Diabetes-friendly foods not only can help control blood sugar levels, but some of them can even repair beta cells and can increase your insulin sensitivity. With regular consumption of these foods, your body naturally builds a defense system against diabetes, and you control diabetes without medicines or with a reduced dose of your medications.

Now let's see which are the top 10 best foods that can help you prevent and control diabetes without medicines.

1.3

10 BEST FOODS TO PREVENT AND CONTROL DIABETES

10 best foods to prevent and control diabetes

Below are 10 best foods to prevent and control diabetes:

1. Bitter gourd (bitter melon)

Bitter gourd (bitter melon) contains compounds that help lower blood glucose and fats levels in the body. Bitter gourd juice is an excellent beverage for people with diabetes. In fact, it is more effective than some second-line drugs for controlling glucose levels in the body. It works through various mechanisms to lower blood sugar levels. It limits the breakdown of the carbohydrates into glucose by inhibiting the carbohydrates metabolizing enzymes.

Furthermore, bitter gourd enhances the glucose uptake by tissues and increases glucose metabolism. It repairs damaged beta cells that make insulin and prevents their death. It contains chemical compounds such as charantin and polypeptide-p that exhibit a hypoglycemic effect. Polypeptide-p or p-insulin is an insulin-like protein. It works by mimicking the action of insulin in the body and very effective in controlling sugar levels in patients with type-1 diabetes.

Bitter gourd helps in treating obesity by boosting the system and enzymes responsible for converting fat into energy. It prevents the accumulation of fat in the body, which prevents fat-induced insulin resistance. In season, you must eat at least one medium bitter gourd or 50-100 ml of bitter gourd juice in a day. Bitter gourd could be your magic pill to reduce your dependence on your anti-diabetic medications. If you are healthy and young but have a family history of diabetes, then you should start eating bitter gourd to prevent diabetes in the future.

2. Fenugreek seeds

Fenugreek seeds are the second most effective food, after bitter gourd to control diabetes naturally. Regular consumption of fenugreek seeds effectively prevents the development of diabetes. Fenugreek seeds increase glucose-induced insulin release. The research finding shows that after consumption of fenugreek seeds soaked in hot water, significantly decrease fasting blood sugar, triglyceride, and LDL-cholesterol up to 30%. If you have diabetes, you should eat fenugreek seeds every day. But before you start eating them, consult your doctor because regular consumption of fenugreek seed decreases your blood sugar levels, and you need a lesser dose of your prescribed drug. Soak fenugreek seeds in a cup of water overnight. The next morning on an empty stomach, chew the seeds and drink the water in which the seeds were soaked.

3. Bottle gourd/Calabash

Consumption of bottle gourd helps reduce blood sugar levels. Bottle gourd is very low in calories and high in both soluble and insoluble dietary fiber. It contains almost 90% water, which makes it a choice of vegetable in diabetes. Bottle gourd helps prevent the development of insulin resistance in type 2 diabetes. It inhibits the action of an enzyme called protein-tyrosine phosphatase (PTP) 1B, which improves glucose metabolism and enhances insulin sensitivity without causing lipid accumulation in the liver and thus helps in obesity control.

Make sure you don't eat bitter bottle gourd. First taste a piece of bottle gourd before cooking, discard it if it is bitter because bitter bottle gourd is not edible and can even cause toxicity and stomach ulcer.

4. Barley

If you want to prevent diabetes, start eating barley regularly. The lower consumption of dietary fiber is associated with the increasing prevalence of diabetes. Barley is an excellent source of soluble fiber along with antioxidant minerals such as magnesium, copper, selenium, and chromium. Research shows long term consumption of barley is effective in lowering blood glucose levels by mimicking the mechanism of action of your first line anti-diabetes drugs. It decreases insulin resistance and interferes with carbohydrates absorption and metabolism. Carbohydrates in barley convert into glucose gradually, without rapidly increasing blood glucose levels. It increases a hormone that helps reduce chronic low-grade inflammation. Barley is an incredible preventive food for those who are at high risk for developing diabetes. You can grind barley and make flour. Add barley flour in wheat flour whenever you make chapati or bread; you can even add barley flour to your cake batter.

5. Monounsaturated fats

Monounsaturated fats such as olive oil, canola oil, and avocado can be advantageous for those with type 1 or type 2 diabetes who are trying to lose or maintain weight. High-monounsaturated-fat diets cause a modest increase in HDL-cholesterol levels, and lower LDL-cholesterol levels, as well as improve glycemic control. Oil containing monounsaturated fats is the choice of oil in diabetes, so choose your cooking oil accordingly. You can protect your heart by replacing saturated fats in your diet with monounsaturated fats. Regular consumption of monounsaturated fats prevents insulin resistance and accumulation of abdominal fat by increasing your fat-burning hormone adiponectin. Keep in mind that oils are high in calories, even the healthiest oils, so consume them in moderation. Your objective should be to replace saturated fats with monounsaturated fats. Keep the intake of polyunsaturated fats (soybean oil, sunflower oil, and corn oil) less than 10% of total energy consumption. Your total fat consumption should be less than 35% of total energy consumption (from carbohydrates and protein).

6. Legumes

Legumes are a superfood for people with diabetes. Legumes such as chickpeas, kidney beans, and peas help manage and reduce type 2 diabetes risk. They are low on the glycemic index (GI) scale despite containing carbohydrates. They increase serum adiponectin concentrations in type 2 diabetic patients that help in preventing abdominal fat and reduce the risk of insulin resistance. Always choose dried beans over canned beans because lots of salt is added in canned products, which can increase your risk of high blood pressure. If you must use canned beans, be sure to rinse them to get rid of salt as much as possible.

7. Zinc

Zinc plays an antioxidant role in type 2 diabetes. It improves oxidative stress by reducing chronic hyperglycemia. It has been seen that people with diabetes have lower levels of zinc than people without diabetes. Zinc deficiency may lead to the development of diabetes. It is because zinc plays a crucial part in insulin metabolism; it helps in the production and secretion of insulin. As zinc strengthens the immune system, it protects beta cells from destruction.

Moreover, zinc prevents diabetes by increasing the levels of adiponectin hormone in the body that helps reduce weight. Studies suggest zinc-rich foods help lower blood sugar levels in type 1 as well as type 2 diabetes. Foods that are high in zinc are cashew nuts, sesame seeds, chickpeas, kidney beans, milk, and oats.

8. Fruits

Because of the sugar content, generally, people with diabetes avoid fruits, which is not right. Fruits are full of soluble fiber and don't contain free sugar that is found in chocolate, cakes, biscuits, fruit juices, and cold drinks. So, if you want to cut down the sugar intake, avoid fruit juices, sugary drinks, and cakes than whole fruits. You can easily have one large banana or a medium apple or one slice of papaya in a day.

9. Low-fat yogurt

Probiotics help to reduce inflammation in the body. Yogurt is the best example of probiotics. Yogurt is low in carbohydrates and contains a good amount of protein, vitamin D, calcium, and potassium. It reduces fasting blood glucose, blood pressure, lipid profile, and other cardiovascular risk factors in people with type 2 diabetes. Probiotics control the glycemic condition by lowering insulin resistance and decreasing the production of inflammatory markers. People who eat yogurt have better control over blood sugar in comparison to those who do not eat yogurt. Choose low-fat yogurt over regular yogurt to prevent weight gain.

10. Indian gooseberry/ Amla

The Indian gooseberry is the richest source of vitamin C, containing 20 times more vitamin C than that of orange. Vitamin C lowers blood pressure in people with type 2 diabetes and protects your heart. Indian gooseberry is rich in nutrients and phytochemicals, such as gallic acid, ellagic acid, gallotannin, and corilagin. These all are potent antioxidants. Through their free radical scavenging properties, these phytochemicals help prevent and control hyperglycemia, cardiac complications, and diabetic complications like nephropathy and neuropathy. Amla favorably impacts on the lipid profile, it significantly elevates HDL-cholesterol and lowers LDL-cholesterol levels. Eat it raw or make chutney or simply boil and consume the strained amla juice.

CONCLUSION

Type 2 diabetes is a lifestyle disease. The best part is you can prevent and control diabetes by making some lifestyle modifications. Lack of awareness and over-promotion of unhealthy foods and bad lifestyle choices are the reason why the incidence of diabetes is increasing in population. There is no harm in enjoying unhealthy foods, considering you are consuming them in moderation. Whether or not your blood sugar level is high, to effectively prevent diabetes, reduce your frequency of eating out. Eat homemade foods. Make every unhealthy food at home, and make it from scratch. By the end, when your food will be ready to eat, you will involuntarily fill with the guilt of eating so many unhealthy things at a time. From the next time, you will crave less. Try this trick, it works!

If you are on diabetes medications, consult your doctor and pharmacist before adding the foods mentioned above in your diet. They can provide you the best advice about which foods you can eat and which ones not, given your diabetes condition and the complications of your diabetes. When you eat the foods mentioned above, your blood glucose levels drop, and you need a lesser dose of medicines. So, regularly discuss with your doctor to adjust the dose accordingly, sometimes doctors just repeat the previous prescription in a hurry without checking your current blood sugar levels.

KEY POINTS

✓ Regularly check your blood pressure. Maintain blood pressure <130/80 mm Hg. Tight control of blood pressure can be more effective than glycemic control in preventing heart disease.

✓ Be active. Play outdoor games, use stairs, don't sit for long. A sedentary lifestyle leads to obesity, which causes insulin resistance.

✓ Increase adiponectin (fat burning hormone) levels in your body by eating monounsaturated fats.

✓ Don't just add additional monounsaturated fats in your diet, instead replace saturated fats with monounsaturated fats.

✓ Drink plenty of water. Water helps remove excess sugar from your blood through urine.

✓ Eat foods that contain soluble fiber and complex carbohydrates that are low in the glycemic index. You can typically eat protein, but proteins are restricted in people who have or are at risk of kidney damage.

✓ Keep an eye on your hypoglycemia symptoms. Always keep some glucose tablets with you.

✓ If you have diabetes, avoid diabetes complications by getting regular diabetes tests, which can catch problems early and can help you prevent serious diabetes complications. Get a yearly eye exam to ensure no blood vessels of the retina has damaged. Get your cholesterol levels checked. Get a regular urine microalbumin tests to check your kidneys' health, and, electrocardiogram to check your heart health.

2

HYPERTENSION

2.1

EVERYTHING YOU NEED TO KNOW ABOUT HYPERTENSION

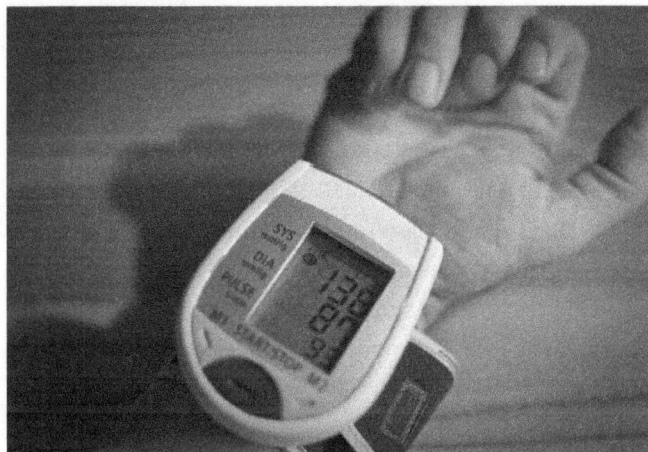

Everything you need to know about hypertension

Hypertension is also known as high blood pressure, is a medical condition that can increase your risk of heart disease, stroke, and other severe health complications. The heart pumps blood into arteries (blood vessels) that carry blood away from the heart to the tissues and organs of the body. Blood pressure is the measure of the force of blood against blood vessel walls. When the force of the blood against the artery walls is too high, it increases the blood pressure, and this condition is known as hypertension.

It is dangerous and needs to be controlled because high blood pressure makes the heart work harder to pump blood out to the organs. This can result in hardening of the arteries (atherosclerosis), stroke, kidney disease, and heart failure.

Blood pressure is expressed by two measurements, maximum and minimum pressures, or a top number and bottom number. Let's see what these numbers are:

Systolic blood pressure - Top number (maximum pressure) tells your systolic pressure. When the heartbeats, it contracts and pumps blood through the arteries to the rest of the body, the contraction creates pressure on blood vessels. This is called systolic blood pressure. Normal systolic pressure is below 120 millimeters of mercury (mm Hg). A reading of 130 mm Hg or higher means high blood pressure.

Diastolic blood pressure - Bottom number (minimum pressure) tells your diastolic pressure. The heart contracts to pump blood to the rest of the body and relaxes before it

110

contracts again. The resting time between beats is when your heart fills with blood and gets oxygen. Diastolic pressure is the pressure of the blood in the arteries when the heart is filling. Normal diastolic pressure is below 80 millimeters of mercury (mm Hg). A reading of 80 mm Hg or higher means high blood pressure.

Among both the numbers, systolic blood pressure is more important than diastolic blood pressure because systolic blood pressure gives the best idea of your risk of having a heart attack or a stroke.

CLASSIFICATION OF BLOOD PRESSURE

Classification of blood pressure for adults aged 18 and older as per ACC/AHA (American College of Cardiology and American Heart Association) and ESC/ESH (European Society of Cardiology and the European Society of Hypertension).

As per ACC/AHA			As per ESC/ESH		
Category	Systolic (mmHg)	Diastolic (mmHg)	Category	Systolic (mmHg)	Diastolic (mmHg)
Normal	Less than 120	Less than 80	Optimal	Less than 120	Less than 80
Elevated	120-129	Less than 80	Normal	120-129	80-84
			High normal	130-139	85-89
Hypertension stage 1	130-139	80-89	Hypertension Grade 1	140-159	90-99
Hypertension stage 2	Equal or more than 140	Equal or more than 90	Hypertension Grade 2	160-179	100-109
			Hypertension Grade 3	Equal or more than 180	Equal or more than 180

As per **ESC/ESH** blood pressure level, **140/90 mm Hg** count as hypertension, whereas new guidelines of **ACC/AHA** count **130/80 mm Hg** as hypertension. It is because of a new study that has found that blood pressure levels between 130/80 mm Hg to 139/89 mm Hg is enough to cause substantial heart and blood vessel complications.

SYMPTOMS OF HIGH BLOOD PRESSURE

In high blood pressure, it is quite possible that you won't experience any symptoms for years or even decades, this is the reason why hypertension count as a silent killer. However, once blood pressure reaches in hypertension stage, a person may have the following symptoms:

- Severe headache (specifically on the back of the head in the morning)

- Chest pain

- Shortness of breath

- Fatigue and confusion

- Vision problems

- Blood in the urine

- Flushing

- Pounding in your chest or neck

The best way to determine whether your blood pressure is high or not is to voluntarily ask your doctor to check your BP when you go for a health check-up. You should get your BP checked every four months. If your blood pressure is elevated, do get checked every month. If you have high blood pressure and you are on medicines, you should check your BP twice a day. The first measurement should be in the morning before eating or taking any medications, and the second in the evening. Each time you measure, take two or three readings at an interval of 1 or 2 mins to make sure your results are accurate.

Let's first understand what actually happens in the body that causes blood pressure to rise.

MECHANISMS THROUGH WHICH BLOOD PRESSURE RISES

1. Abnormalities of the sympathetic nervous system

You must have heard it many times "*do not stress, or else your blood pressure will go up*," and it's absolutely right." The sympathetic nervous system influences the blood vessels of the body in a dangerous or stressful condition. When you stress out, sympathetic outflow increases. The sympathetic nervous system release the hormones adrenaline and noradrenaline (also known as norepinephrine). These hormones increase the rate of blood pumping from the heart to deliver fresh oxygen to the brain and muscles. The repeated stress means a continuous increase in blood pumping from the heart, which is attained by constricting the blood vessels. The constant constriction of the blood vessels causes the narrowing of the blood vessels and increases the resistance of the blood vessels to blood flow (peripheral resistance). As a result, blood pressure increases.

2. Abnormalities in the intrarenal renin-angiotensin-aldosterone system (RAAS)

This system controls blood pressure by regulating the volume of fluids in the body. When blood flow to the kidneys decreases, the kidneys secrete enzyme renin into blood circulation. Plasma renin then converts angiotensinogen to angiotensin I, which have no direct biological activity. However, an enzyme known as Angiotensin-Converting Enzyme (ACE) converts Angiotensin I to Angiotensin II (the primary hormone responsible for high blood pressure). Angiotensin II is a peptide hormone that causes vasoconstriction, which means it contracts the muscular wall of the vessels, which causes the narrowing of the blood vessels, resulting in increased blood pressure.

RISK FACTORS

Below are the contributory factors that increase your blood pressure:

- Stress
- Obesity
- Excess alcohol
- Smoking

- Family history of high blood pressure

- Excess salt intake

- A diet lack of potassium

- Lack of exercise

- Certain drugs such as NSAIDs, steroids and contraceptive pills

WHY IS HYPERTENSION DANGEROUS?

Hypertension or High Blood Pressure is dangerous because it causes other health complications. Blood vessels are responsible for delivering oxygen and nutrients to vital organs and tissues. Over time, high blood pressure damages the blood vessels. The damaged blood vessels disrupt the blood flow in the body that cause other health problems to arise. The most affected part of the body by hypertension is heart, followed by, brain, kidney, and reproductive system.

Heart attack   Dementia

Hypertension complications

Kidney failure   Brain stroke

Blurred vision

Damage to the arteries

Blood vessels that carry oxygen-rich blood from the heart to the body are called arteries. Arteries are flexible, elastic, and their inner lining is smooth. Blood flows freely and unobstructed through healthy arteries and supply oxygen and nutrients to vital organs and tissues. High blood pressure reduces the elasticity of arteries. It damages their inner lining that makes it easier for dietary fats to collect in the damaged arteries, limiting blood flow throughout your body. These blockages eventually can lead to heart attack and stroke.

Damage to the heart

Hypertension makes your heart pump more frequently, and with more force than a healthy heart, which causes part of your heart (left ventricle) to thicken. An enlarged heart increases your risk of heart attack, heart failure, and sudden cardiac death.

Also, high blood pressure damages the vessels that supply blood to your heart. When blood flow to your heart is obstructed, it can cause arrhythmia (irregular heart rhythms), angina (chest pain), or can cause a heart attack.

Damage to the brain

Our brain depends on nourishing oxygen-rich blood supply to work properly. But high blood pressure can reduce blood and oxygen supply to the brain that can cause several problems, including:

Transient Ischemic Attack (TIA): Hardened arteries or blood clots caused by high blood pressure can temporarily disrupt the blood supply to the brain, which is called a transient ischemic attack (TIA) or mini-stroke. TIA count as a warning of a full-blown stroke.

Stroke: High blood pressure can cause blood clots to form in the arteries, leading to significant blockages in blood flow. Reduced blood flow makes the brain deprived of oxygen and nutrients, causing brain cells to die. This is known as a stroke.

Dementia: Certain types of dementia, such as vascular dementia, is caused by a lack of blood flow in the brain, which may have caused by narrowed/blocked arteries or due to a stroke.

Damage to the kidneys

Kidneys filter excess fluid and waste from the blood. High blood pressure damages the blood vessels in and leading to your kidneys. Damaged vessels obstruct the blood flow to the kidneys and prevent kidneys from effectively filtering waste from your blood, allowing dangerous waste to accumulate. Hypertension is one of the most common causes of kidney failure.

Damage to the eyes

High blood pressure can damage the blood vessels that supply blood to your eyes. Limited blood flow can damage the retina and the optic nerve, leading to bleeding in the eye, blurred vision, and even complete loss of vision.

MECHANISM THROUGH WHICH ANTI-HYPERTENSIVE MEDICINES WORK

The primary purpose of all the anti-hypertensive drugs is to produce vasodilation means to make the blood vessels wider or more open. When blood vessels dilate, blood freely flows through them, causing a fall in blood pressure.

There are different mechanisms through which different classes of drugs achieve vasodilation. Let's see in brief how do these drugs work and how can we produce similar effect through foods, which are safer and have no side effects:

The first-line therapy or most common drugs that are used in hypertension lower the blood pressure by decreasing the salt reabsorption in the kidneys. That means your body now has less salt because more and more salt, along with water, are flushed out from the body through urine. Because you have less fluid in your blood vessels, the pressure inside will be lower. The drugs that work on this mechanism are called Diuretics. Our aim is to include foods that naturally have a diuretic effect. We will later see in detail about the foods that are natural diuretics.

As we discussed above, the Angiotensin II hormone is the main culprit behind high blood pressure. So, the other class of drugs produces vasodilation either by blocking the conversion of angiotensin I to angiotensin II (ACE inhibitors drugs) or by blocking the actions of angiotensin II (Angiotensin receptor blockers drugs). This allows blood vessels to widen and relax, making it easier for blood to flow through, which lowers your blood pressure.

Calcium stimulates the heart to contract more forcefully. A class of drugs called calcium channel blockers limits the rate at which calcium flows into the cells of the heart and blood vessel walls. As a result, blood vessels widen, and your heart doesn't have to work as hard to pump, making it easier for blood to flow through, and your blood pressure lowers.

STRATEGY TO PREVENT AND CONTROL HYPERTENSION

Hypertension is food and lifestyle-related disease that means foods play the most significant part in correcting as well as worsening the condition. Hypertension cannot be solely managed with medicines. Certain diet and lifestyle modifications are must for controlling the disease effectively. Medications prescribed in hypertension have side effects that include erectile impotence, gout, cough, and lack of energy. By adding the right foods for high blood pressure in your diet and avoiding the bad foods, you can effectively lower your blood pressure and can drastically reduce the dose of your blood pressure medicines.

Below are certain ways by which you can lower your blood pressure naturally:

- Eat foods that reduce sodium levels in the body.

- Exclude foods that silently add salt in your body.

- Eat foods that are naturally diuretic.

- Eat foods that reduce fluid retention in the body and increase urine production.

- Eat foods that are rich in magnesium as magnesium is a natural calcium channel blocker.

- Eat foods that are rich in potassium because potassium negates the sodium effect.

- Eat foods rich in nitrates, which convert into nitric oxide in your body. Nitric oxide widens the blood vessels and lowers blood pressure.

- By increasing water intake.

SALT

It must have come to your mind that why is it said to avoid table salt in hypertension? What is the exact relationship between salt and blood pressure? So, let's see why salt is dangerous for blood pressure.

Sodium is the main reason for rising blood pressure, and your table salt is basically a combination of sodium

(40%) and chloride (60%). Are salt and sodium the same? No, not exactly. Sodium is a mineral that occurs naturally in foods. With table salt, you eat sodium in the form of sodium chloride. This is the reason why table salt considered dangerous for high blood pressure.

Other forms of sodium that you consume are

Sodium bicarbonate (baking soda) and

Monosodium glutamate (MSG): Generally used as salt in Chinese foods.

HOW DOES SALT INCREASE BLOOD PRESSURE?

Eating salt raises the amount of sodium in your bloodstream. It affects the performance of your kidneys to remove the water. As a result, your body holds extra water to flush out the extra sodium from your body. This is called fluid retention. The excess fluid in the body puts stress on blood vessels and heart and causes blood pressure to rise.

2.2

10 FOODS THAT RAISE YOUR BLOOD PRESSURE

10 foods that raise your blood pressure

Foods that are high in calories increase cholesterol in your body, which raises blood pressure. Some foods silently add salt to your body and increase your risk of high blood pressure. You don't even release that you are eating salt.

To help you identify these foods, here's a list of 10 foods and drinks that knowingly or silently add salt and cholesterol in your body and can raise your blood pressure.

1. Canned foods or beverages

Canned food products are prepared with lots of salt to preserve the food from decaying, and for taste. This decreases the nutrition of the food and silently add salt in your body. For example, as such, chickpeas are very nutritious and have great health benefits, but if you are using canned chickpeas, then they are harmful to your health. Whenever possible, eat fresh foods instead of canned ones. Even if you are using canned chickpeas or other canned vegetables, wash them properly before use to remove the extra salt. Cans are often lined with the chemical bisphenol A (BPA). Eating foods from cans lined with the chemical bisphenol A (BPA) could raise your blood pressure.

2. Deep-fried foods

Eating deep-fried foods, such as french fries, bagels, and puris, increases your risk of high blood pressure, heart attack, and stroke. Fried foods add a lot of calories and deficient in healthy nutrients. These increase cholesterol levels in the body and raise your blood pressure. You should never reuse the oil that has been used in deep frying, also don't fry at high temperature. When you deep fry, oils break down with each frying, and their composition changes. As a result, a chemical is formed in food that can lead to cancer.

3. Pickles

Eating pickles can raise your blood pressure. Lots of salt and oil are required for preserving pickles for long. Salt and oil stop the food from decaying and keep them edible for long. Adding extra sodium of pickle to your diet causes water retention that puts greater pressure on blood vessels and increases blood pressure. Furthermore, pickles are loaded with excess oil that can increase cholesterol in your body. Cholesterol can narrow the blood vessels that prevent the free-flowing of blood and make it harder for the heart to pump blood through them. As a result, your blood pressure rises.

4. Processed cheese

Processed cheese is high on calories and salt. This means regular consumption can lead to high cholesterol, obesity, and high blood pressure, increasing your risk of heart disease. Avoid eating too much-processed cheese. Instead of processed cheese, go for homemade cottage cheese. You can even eat mozzarella cheese as it contains the lowest salt in comparison to other varieties. Cheese can offer health benefits as they are rich in calcium and vitamins. However, if you have diagnosed with high blood pressure, avoid eating any cheese except homemade low-fat cottage cheese (not the store-bought).

5. Caffeine

Your one cup of coffee may give a boost to start your day in an active mode, but it is not good for blood pressure. Caffeine increases the release of the hormone adrenaline, which is responsible for making you active within some minutes of consumption. However, this same hormone adrenaline causes constriction of blood vessels and increases the rate and force of heart pumping. As a result, pressure inside your blood vessels increases. Don't quit tea or coffee completely, instead gradually reduce the frequency, and soon your body will adapt it. Quitting the caffeine all of a sudden will only make you more crave for it.

6. Dehydration

Keep yourself hydrated. When your body is dehydrated, your brain sends a signal to the pituitary gland to secrete hormone vasopressin, which is an antidiuretic hormone. It constricts the blood vessels. As a result, pressure inside the blood vessels increases, which leads to hypertension. Drink at least eight glasses of water in a day. Drinking enough water in pregnancy is essential, especially if your blood pressure is already high, to prevent toxemia, which is a potentially dangerous pregnancy complication characterized by the onset of high blood pressure.

7. Smoking

Each cigarette you smoke increases your blood pressure. The nicotine in cigarettes is the main reason for high blood pressure. Nicotine stimulates the central nervous system. High blood pressure is caused by both an increase in cardiac output and total peripheral vascular resistance. Nicotine acts as a stimulant in the body. It stimulates the adrenal glands to release more adrenaline. It forces the heart to constrict more forcefully, which affects the heart pumping capacity. It narrows your blood vessels and hardens their walls. As a result, your blood flow gets restricted, which increases peripheral vascular resistance and makes your blood more likely to clot. If you smoke, quit it as soon as possible—people who quit smoking live longer than people who smoke.

8. Alcohol

Any alcoholic beverage can increase your blood pressure. Alcohol interferes with the effectiveness of your anti-hypertensive drugs. In fact, even one drink can change the way your blood pressure medications work and increase the side effects of blood pressure medications. Alcohol increases blood pressure by increasing cortisol (stress hormone) levels. Alcohol stimulates the release of vasoconstrictor angiotensin II and induces inflammation that inhibits nitric oxide production in the body. Alcohol is high in calories and may contribute to unwanted weight gain, which is a risk factor for high blood pressure. If you want to prevent high blood pressure, quit drinking completely.

9. Sugar

It might surprise you, but high sugar intake is linked with hypertension. Not only because it leads to obesity, but it causes high blood pressure through a different mechanism too. Sugar elevates uric acid in the body that induces oxidative stress and decreases endothelial nitric oxide availability. It also activates both renin activity and angiotensin activity in the kidney. Nitric oxide suppression, as well as enhancement of angiotensin activity, constricts the blood vessels, leading to high blood pressure. Sugar also gives empty calories and increases cholesterol in the body. Increased cholesterol causes plaque to build up inside your arteries, and arteries become hardened and narrowed. As a result, your heart has to work much harder to pump blood through them and cause an increase in your blood pressure.

10. Packaged snacks

Potato chips, popcorns, sev, banana chips, and other packaged snacks have lots of salt in it. More the flavors, the more the salt content. Flavors like salted, cream, and onion have more salt content. Additionally, these are high in saturated and trans fats, sugar, and other low-fiber carbohydrates. Consuming too much of packaged snacks increases bad cholesterol (LDL) in the body. High LDL levels may lead to the formation of cholesterol plaque in the blood vessel that constricts the free-flowing of blood and may eventually lead to the development of coronary heart disease. You don't need to stop eating snacks completely, but do limit your servings and frequency. Look for plain version instead of flavored.

2.3

10 FOODS THAT LOWER BLOOD PRESSURE JUST LIKE ANTIHYPERTENSIVE DRUGS

10 foods that lower blood pressure just like antihypertensive drugs

Certain foods naturally lower blood pressure. Adding these foods in your diet can significantly reduce your risk of high blood pressure. A diet low in sodium and rich in potassium, magnesium, nitrate, and fiber can help prevent and control blood pressure.

Below are the top 10 foods that work just like antihypertensive drugs and lower your blood pressure:

1. Leafy green vegetables

Leafy green vegetables such as spinach, kale, fennel, and cabbage are very dense in nutrition. These are packed with potassium, magnesium, nitrates, and full of fiber. Low potassium intake is one of the risk factors in developing high blood pressure. The potassium content of leafy green vegetables flushes out sodium. The rich magnesium content act as calcium channel antagonist, modulating vascular tone and reactivity that dilates blood vessels. As a result, blood flows without any restriction through your blood vessels, and your blood pressure decreases.

Moreover, nitrate of leafy greens induces vasodilation. Nitrate converts into nitrite in your mouth by oral commensal bacteria. It then converts in nitric oxide in your blood, which relaxes the smooth muscle of your blood vessels and dilates them that allows free-flowing of blood. Prevent using antibacterial mouthwash as it inhibits nitrate to nitrite conversion, and you don't get the blood pressure-lowering benefit of nitric oxide.

2. Beetroot

Beetroot is a well-known potent vasodilator. It contains high levels of dietary nitrate; the body converts the nitrate in this vegetable into nitric oxide. Nitric oxide relaxes and dilates blood vessels, so lowering blood pressure. For the full benefit, drink a glass of raw beetroot juice because raw beetroot has more potency than cooked one. Research indicates that within hours of drinking raw beetroot juice, it lowers systolic blood pressure.

3. Garlic

Eating garlic every day may help reduce your blood pressure. The organosulfur compounds of garlic promote vasodilation and lower blood pressure. Garlic lowers blood pressure through various mechanisms of action. Dietary intake of garlic boosts hydrogen sulfide production and regulation of endothelial nitric oxide, which induces smooth muscle cell relaxation and vasodilation; as a result, blood pressure drops. Garlic also blocks angiotensin-II production by inhibition of the angiotensin-converting-enzyme (ACE).

Allicin is an organosulfur compound that releases when garlic is crushed or chopped. Allicin is highly unstable. Cooking speeds up the degradation of allicin, and microwaving destroys it completely.

Eat one clove of freshly crushed garlic empty stomach every day, and it will lower your blood pressure naturally. But keep in mind that raw garlic is quite pungent and can cause burn, so don't hold it in your mouth for long periods. Too much garlic may cause irritation and digestive upset. If you see the irritation, limit the frequency to 2 to 3 times a week.

4. Cucumber

Cucumber is rich in potassium, which plays an important role in regulating blood pressure. The excess sodium in your body reduces the ability of your kidneys to remove the water. This makes your body hold fluids that raises your blood pressure. Potassium lowers blood pressure by balancing out the adverse effects of sodium. The more potassium you eat, the more sodium you lose through urine. Also, cucumber is a diuretic. It flushes out sodium from the body by increasing your urine production and maintain fluid balance in the body that helps keep blood pressure in check. Use cucumber in salad, raita, or have cucumber juice.

5. Banana

What can be a better source of potassium than the well-known and probably most blood pressure friendly fruit banana! Eating potassium-rich foods decrease sodium levels in your body. It reduces fluid retention and blood pressure by increasing urine production. Potassium also acts as a vasodilator that helps ease tension in your blood vessel walls, which helps lower blood pressure. Banana is one of the healthiest fruits because it is very low in calories and has higher water content.

6. Lemon water

Lemon is an excellent remedy for hypertension as it helps keep blood vessels soft and pliable, making them flexible by removing any rigidity. This keeps the blood pressure low. Lemon is rich in vitamin C that works as an antioxidant and has a diuretic effect. It removes excess fluid from your body, which lowers the blood pressure. Furthermore, vitamin C helps protect the levels of nitric oxide in the body that relaxes blood vessels and contributes to maintaining normal and healthy blood pressure. Taking a glass of warm lemon water every morning on an empty stomach helps you keep the high blood pressure at bay. If you are on blood pressure medicines, do consult your doctor and pharmacist before including citrus fruits like lemon in your diet as citrus fruits can interact with your medications, especially calcium antagonist drugs.

7. Honey

Honey contains antioxidant compounds that are linked to lower blood pressure. Obesity and unhealthy lifestyle cause oxidative stress in your body that reduces vasodilatory agent nitric oxide available in the body. The antioxidants present in honey help to keep the nitric oxide levels high in the body by reducing oxidative stress in the body. Nitric oxide relaxes your blood vessels causing vasodilation, which helps to lower the blood pressure. Take one tablespoon of honey daily or add it in your morning lemon water. Make sure you eat organic honey, not the processed ones. Eat it raw, don't heat the honey. Heating honey destroys the beneficial enzymes, vitamins, and minerals of the honey.

8. Nuts

Nuts such as almonds, cashew nuts, and walnuts are rich in magnesium, fiber, and protein. Magnesium is an electrolyte that helps lower high blood pressure. Magnesium is a natural calcium channel blocker, it stimulates the production of vasodilators nitric oxide and prostacyclins. These vasodilators relax the blood vessels and lower blood pressure. Nuts also contain heart-healthy fats that lower cholesterol levels. Remember to get magnesium from your food, not from supplements, to avoid any risk of overdose. Make sure to eat nuts every day.

9. Fenugreek seeds

Drinking fenugreek water can be one of the most effective ways for you to maintain healthy blood pressure. Fenugreek leaves and seeds contain a high amount of dietary fiber. A diet rich in fiber has been linked to steady levels of blood pressure. Dietary fiber is tough to digest. It forms a viscous gel in the intestine that makes it harder for sugars and fats to absorb in the bloodstream and decreases cholesterol levels in the body and prevent weight gain. Furthermore, fenugreek leaves and seeds contain low levels of sodium, which makes it an ideal food for people with high blood pressure.

Take two teaspoons of fenugreek seeds and soak them in a glass of water overnight. The next morning remove the seeds from water, drink the fenugreek water on an empty stomach. Crush the seeds to a fine paste and use it in cooking. Do this for at least two to three months and see the positive result yourself.

10. legumes

Legumes such as lentils, chickpeas, kidney beans, soybeans, and others, are rich in potassium, magnesium, and fiber. These nutrients maintain healthy and normal blood pressure. Potassium and magnesium in legumes prevent fluid retention, decrease sodium levels by increasing urine production. The soluble fiber in the legumes gets attached to cholesterol particles and takes them out of the body that helps to reduce overall cholesterol levels. This reduces the risk of weight gain and improves vascular health.

IMPLEMENTATION

Now that you know everything about hypertension, how blood pressure works, what exactly goes wrong in your body in hypertension condition, what are the risk factors, what you should avoid and what you should start adding in your diet? Now the question arises, how to implement it?

If you are a healthy person and have no hypertension condition and no family history of hypertension, start with adding foods in your diet that can help you prevent hypertension in the future. Start with adding above mentioned foods that are most of your likening, gradually add those foods in your diet that you do not like much but make sure to add them, gradually you will be habitual. You must add sweet potato, onion, and pomegranate too in your diet; these foods are also very effective in preventing high blood pressure. Limit your consumption of food that increases your risk of high blood pressure. If you smoke, quit it. Limit your alcohol consumption.

If you are a healthy person but have a family history of hypertension, strictly avoid eating known and silent salt-rich foods. With a family history of hypertension, you are susceptible to high blood pressure. Quit smoking and drinking any alcoholic beverages completely, don't increase your risk of high blood pressure. Eat foods as mentioned above that naturally prevent hypertension, also include sweet potato, pomegranate in your diet, but if you have a family history of diabetes too, then limit your consumption of sugar as well as sweet fruits.

If you are a person with high blood pressure, you must eat potassium-rich foods. The best way is to note down all the above mentioned preventive foods, ask your doctor and pharmacist:

I want to add these foods in my diet, is it safe to add all of them? Are there any foods that can interact with my medications? They will provide you the best advice considering your blood pressure levels and other health complications. Let them know if you have other health problems like diabetes and arthritis. If you have diabetes, then limit the consumption of high glycemic foods. If you have arthritis, limit your citrus fruit consumption. After including these foods for three months, ask your doctor, has my blood pressure improved? Do I need the same dose of medicines or lower dose will work? Keep in mind once you have controlled your blood pressure, continue to consume foods that prevent high blood pressure. It should be a lifetime habit, not short-term therapy.

KEY POINTS

✓ Consume less salt. It promotes fluid retention that increases blood pressure.

✓ Avoid foods that silently add salt in your body.

✓ Eat foods low in fat and calories.

✓ Do yoga.

✓ Be active. Physical activity reduces water retention by making you sweat and increasing blood flow to the tissues.

✓ Drink plenty of water, especially on the day you consume more salt. Dehydration can increase your risk of water retention.

✓ Don't stress out.

✓ Eat whole grains instead of refined ones.

✓ Add barley flour to your whole wheat flour in a ratio of 2:10. Add 200 gm of barley flour to 1 kg of whole wheat flour.

3

ARTHRITIS

3.1

EVERYTHING YOU NEED TO KNOW ABOUT ARTHRITIS

Everything you need to know about arthritis

To prevent any disease, first, you need to understand that disease, how that particular disease affects your body, how your body is reacting to disease. What are the points to be taken into consideration while managing that disease? In managing any disease, food and lifestyle play an extremely important role. In a disease condition, the damage that has already been done to the body is out of our control. But limiting the disease's spread and reversing its effect is totally on our hands.

So, let's see how to prevent and manage arthritis.

What is arthritis?

It is a joint disorder featuring inflammation with stiffness and joint pain. It can be of one or more joints—a joint means where two different bones meet for the purpose of permitting body parts to move.

Types of Arthritis

There are more than 100 types of arthritis. Two of the most common types are

Osteoarthritis (OA)

Rheumatoid arthritis (RA)

OSTEOARTHRITIS (OA)

The breakdown of cartilage is called Osteoarthritis. Cartilage is the protective hard, slippery tissue that caps the ends of bones where two bones form a joint. Cartilage cushions the ends of the bones and responsible for smooth and frictionless movement. When this protective layer gets damaged, it results in friction between the bones. The continuous friction causes pain and restricts the joint movement. It mainly occurs in the hands, neck, knees, hips, or lower back.

Causes of Osteoarthritis

Injury to joints or ligaments

- Joint infection

- Diabetes

- Obesity

- Low levels of estrogen hormone in women (mainly after menopause)

RHEUMATOID ARTHRITIS (RA)

Rheumatoid arthritis (RA) is a chronic autoimmune disease in which the immune system mistakenly attacks the joints — mainly the lining of joints (called synovium). This results in inflammation of the affected tissues in and around joints. Eventually, inflammation destroys the joint, and joint loses its shape and alignment.

Rheumatoid arthritis symptoms include:

- Joint pain

- Swollen joints

- Joint stiffness, usually in the mornings

- Fatigue

- Fever

- Joint redness

- Joint deformities

Who is prone to rheumatoid arthritis?

Adults over 55 years

Mostly women

Obese people

What do antirheumatic medications do?

RA medications actually don't treat arthritis but slow the damage that arthritis can cause to your body by

Reducing the pain and

Decreasing the inflammation

The pain-relieving nonsteroidal anti-inflammatory drugs (NSAIDs) reduce pain and inflammation by blocking an enzyme called, COX-2 enzyme and reduce the production of prostaglandins. Prostaglandins are chemicals that promote pain, inflammation, swelling, and fever.

While another class of drugs, disease-modifying antirheumatic drugs (DMARDs) slow down the progression of rheumatoid arthritis by reducing the response of the immune system.

The problem with these drugs is that they may have serious side effects. The RA condition can be easily managed with food therapy. Our motive is to include foods in our diet that are natural COX-2 inhibitors and to exclude foods that promote inflammation in the body.

PREVENTION AND CONTROL OF ARTHRITIS THROUGH FOOD

Diet has a massive impact on arthritis conditions. Some foods cause inflammation in the body, either by increasing free radicals in the body or by enhancing the release of pro-inflammatory proteins. You can prevent arthritis by avoiding any food that causes inflammation in the body. But, for that, you must know the types of foods that cause inflammation or aggravate the pain. Similarly, some foods are potent anti-oxidant and anti-inflammatory. These foods are considered as superfoods for arthritis because they act as natural COX-2 inhibitors and prevent inflammation in the body as well as promote the secretion of the anti-inflammatory protein, which reduce inflammation by preventing oxidative stress in the body.

3.2

10 FOODS THAT INCREASE YOUR RISK OF ARTHRITIS OR MAY FLARE UP YOUR ARTHRITIS

10 foods that increase your risk of arthritis or may flare up your arthritis

Any sour food can flare up your arthritis. Many people have complained that certain foods induce arthritis pain. It can differ from person to person. Some people may experience pain, while others have no effects with these foods. You can check it by yourself, how's your body reacting to these foods. If you experience pain with the following foods, then stop taking them one by one for about 1-2 weeks. If the pain and stiffness go away, that means that particular food is flaring up your arthritis. Don't completely stop taking these foods but consume them in moderation.

Here are the foods that may flare up your arthritis:

1 Sunflower oil

Sunflower oil can lead to joint pain and inflammation. Sunflower oil contains omega-6 fatty acids. Arachidonic acid (ARA), a polyunsaturated omega-6 fatty acid triggers the body to produce potent pro-inflammatory mediators such as prostaglandins and leukotrienes that cause inflammation - a key cause of arthritis pain. Polyunsaturated oils contain two types of essential fatty acids, omega-3 fatty acids, and omega-6 fatty acids. Your body itself cannot produce these fatty acids, so you need to get them from food. Omega-3 fats are anti-inflammatory, while omega-6 fats are pro-inflammatory. You need not completely stop taking omega-6 fatty acids. Both are essential for the body, but excess consumption of omega-6 fats is bad for rheumatoid arthritis. Avoid sunflower oil.

2. Sour curd

Freshly made curd in moderation may not be bad for arthritis, but sour curd often aggravates arthritis pain. Casein – a type of protein present in curd promote inflammation, which is the main reason for rheumatoid arthritis. Avoid sour curd; always eat fresh curd made on the same day, that too in moderation.

3. Tamarind

As such, tamarind is very beneficial for health but not for rheumatoid arthritis. This sweet and sour fruit can worsen arthritis pain and inflammation. Although studies suggest tamarind abrogates arthritis-mediated cartilage and bone degradation, but some people experience an increase in pain with tamarind. Again, the experience can differ from person to person; hence it is advised to observe your body's reaction to tamarind.

4. Nightshade vegetables

Both potatoes and eggplants are members of the nightshade family. Both contain the chemical solanine that plants use as a natural defense. It has a toxic effect on the body and can lead to gastrointestinal and neurological disorders. People claim that they experience arthritis pain and inflammation with nightshade vegetables, which can be due to solanine.

Other vegetables from the nightshade family are tomatoes and peppers. If you experience an increase in inflammation and pain after consuming any of these vegetables, avoid them. Even if you don't experience any pain, still eat them in moderation.

5. Black gram

Black gram increases pro-inflammatory cytokines IL-1β and TNF-α and decreases anti-inflammatory cytokine IL-10. It means it increases inflammation in the body by increasing inflammation-causing protein and decreasing the protein that reduces inflammation in the body. Also, research suggests black gram decreases antioxidant effect in the body, which is more prominent in black gram without skin; boiling and not boiling the pulse doesn't have much difference in their effects.

6. Taro root/Arbi

Taro root comprises of calcium oxalate in a needle-shaped crystal form, which can produce irritation and burning sensation when consumed in raw form. Many arthritis people claim that they experience swelling and pain after taro root consumption. They may cause the formation of kidney stones and gout (a type of arthritis), accompanied by some other health issues. Either avoid eating this root or boil the root for an extended period before cooking them.

7. Chilled water

Chilled water can worsen autoimmune diseases, including rheumatoid arthritis. Chilled water causes constriction of blood vessels and reduces blood flow to the affected joint area. Due to reduced blood flow, the body's ability to clear out the impurities gets affected, and inflammation increases resulting in pain. Avoid drinking anything chill, whether it's a cold drink, iced tea, cold coffee, or plain chilled water.

8. Fried foods

When foods are exposed to high temperatures, such as during frying, baking, barbecuing, and grilling, produce advanced glycation end product (AGE), which is a toxin. AGEs bind to RAGE (receptor for advanced glycation end-products) and activate pro-inflammatory cytokine production, thus become involved in inflammation and result in arthritis.

9. Processed foods and canned foods

Canned foods contain excessive salt and other preservatives to achieve longer shelf lives. High sodium can increase inflammation in your body. Reducing salt consumption may help in reducing inflammation. Processed foods such as cakes, biscuit, and cheese contain hydrogenated oils that are high in trans fats, and trans fats trigger systemic inflammation. Avoid processed and canned foods to prevent arthritis.

10. Alcohol

Drinking alcohol is injurious to health; you must have heard it many times. Alcohol may cause more inflammation, which can make symptoms of arthritis worse. Alcohol interferes with anti-inflammatory medicines that can increase your risk of stomach bleeding and ulcers and can be fatal. Never drink if you are on arthritis medication.

155

CONCLUSION

Not everyone reacts the same way to the foods mentioned above. Some can easily tolerate these foods, while others' pain gets worse. You know your body best. Observe yourself. Note down what you eat the whole day and observe if you experience an increase in pain, swelling, and inflammation. If any of the above foods were included in your diet, avoid eating them for about 1 to 2 weeks and see if your condition gets better. Just by avoiding these foods, preventing and managing your arthritis would be much easier. If you are young, healthy, and have no arthritis history in your family, limit your consumption of the foods mentioned above, and arthritis will never touch you in life.

3.3

10 FOODS THAT HELP PREVENT AND CONTROL ARTHRITIS

10 foods that help prevent and control arthritis

To prevent and control arthritis, your diet should be rich in foods that have the following activities:

- Foods that reduce inflammation (omega-3 rich foods)

- Foods that have potent antioxidant property

- Foods that modulate immune activity

- Foods that balance the gut microbiome

Below are the 10 power foods that can prevent and treat arthritis naturally:

1. Horse gram

Horse gram is rich in polyphenols, flavonoids, and acts as an anti-inflammatory and an antioxidant. Studies show that horse gram significantly increases the activity of antioxidant enzymes such as catalase, superoxide dismutase, glutathione peroxidase, in liver and heart. Horse gram decreases inflammation by increasing the levels of anti-inflammatory cytokine IL-10 in the body. Because of the potent anti-inflammatory and antioxidant activities, horse gram can reverse arthritis. Additionally, it helps reduce body weight. Weight loss may help improve arthritis symptoms by reducing the excess load on your joints that cause pain and discomfort.

2. Turmeric

The main active ingredient in turmeric is curcumin. It is curcumin that gives turmeric bright yellow color. It produces potent anti-inflammatory and antioxidant effects. Typical medicines that are prescribed in arthritis are non-steroidal anti-inflammatory drugs (NSAIDs). These drugs work by inhibiting the activity of cyclooxygenase enzymes, COX-1, and COX-2. COX-1 is the good COX, while COX-2 is potentially troublesome. COX-1 synthesizes prostaglandins that help in maintaining the health of the stomach and intestine, while COX-2 synthesizes the inflammatory prostaglandins and oxygen-free radicals that enhance inflammation. These NSAIDs inhibit the COX-2 enzyme, but simultaneously they inhibit the good COX-1 too. Therefore, they may increase the risk of serious bowel and stomach side effects like ulcers and bleeding. Studies suggest curcumin has the chemical properties of a COX inhibitor and has no side effects like NSAIDs. Turmeric may help alleviate or prevent symptoms of arthritis. Turmeric is very effective in preventing arthritis.

Boil one glass of milk and add one tablespoon of turmeric powder in it. Drink it at night just before bed while it's still hot. In winter, eat plenty of fresh turmeric roots. They are more effective and beneficial than turmeric powder.

3. Ginger

Ginger has potent antioxidant and anti-inflammatory properties. It increases the activities of antioxidant enzymes in the liver. Ginger contains phenolic compounds such as gingerol and shogaols as active components that protect body tissues against oxidative stress. Ginger also suppresses the synthesis of pro-inflammatory cytokines by suppressing NF-κB protein. It has been proven that ginger functions as a COX-2 inhibitor, just like NSAIDs, in controlling rheumatoid arthritis, osteoarthritis, and other types of arthritis. The anti-inflammatory properties of ginger help relieve pain and improve conditions in all types of arthritis.

4. Walnuts

Walnuts have excellent antioxidant and anti-inflammatory activity. Phenolic content of walnut, especially in its skin, exhibits the highest ant-oxidative capacity. Walnuts are high in alpha-linolenic acid (ALA). They have the highest omega-3 content in comparison to other tree nuts. Omega-3 fats have anti-inflammatory effects that reduce inflammation. Elevated C-reactive protein (CRP) levels in the body indicate the inflammatory condition like RA. Studies show walnuts lower C-reactive protein (CRP), a marker of inflammation linked to arthritis.

Take a handful of walnut kernels or two whole walnuts, soak them in water overnight. Eat them on an empty stomach the next morning. Soaking is an important step, especially in the summer season, because walnuts are warm in nature. Walnuts can produce heat in the body and can cause mouth ulcers if you consume them without soaking.

5. Extra virgin olive oil

Extra virgin olive oil is rich in Omega-3 fatty acids. Omega-3 fats work as an anti-inflammatory and help reduce pain and swelling in arthritic joints. Alongside Omega-3 fatty acids, olive oil also contains oleocanthal, a natural compound that has scientifically proven to produce similar pain-relieving results as non-steroidal anti-inflammatory drugs (NSAIDs). Oleocanthal works in a similar way to NSAIDs by inhibiting the same enzyme responsible for inflammation and pain. Additionally, phenolic compounds present in extra virgin olive oil reduce cartilage degradation, bone erosion, and joint edema.

Also, a recent study suggests applying topical extra virgin olive oil is effective in controlling of inflammatory pain of joints in rheumatic arthritis.

Among all types of olive oils, extra virgin olive oil exhibits maximum health benefits, because it is the least processed or refined type. It contains maximum phenolic antioxidants and oleocanthal content.

6. Licorice root

Licorice decreases the levels of pro-inflammatory cytokines. Glycyrrhizin is the component in licorice, which exhibits an anti-inflammatory effect by mimicking the actions of steroids in the body. Furthermore, licorice prevents oxidative damages. Licorice increases the availability of cortisol in the body by preventing the body from using up its stores of cortisol; it reduces the conversion of cortisol to inactive cortisone. Cortisol can help reduce inflammation, also, suppresses the immune system, easing the pain and occurrence of arthritis. Be aware that licorice can cause anxiety and high blood pressure. If you are on medication of blood pressure, diabetes or diuretics, don't use licorice, it may interfere with the drug's efficacy. Consult your doctor before taking licorice. Women who are pregnant are not advised to take licorice root in any form. Licorice should be taken under medical advice. Roasting licorice roots increase their anti-inflammatory activity. Research show roasted licorice may inhibit the acute inflammation more potently. The best way to take licorice root is to roast it, crush it and to boil up the root in order to make a herbal tea.

7. Flax seeds

Flax seeds are also known as linseeds. Flax seeds and flax seeds oil are rich in alpha-linolenic acid (ALA), an omega-3 fatty acid that helps decrease inflammation and joint pain in arthritis. Phytochemicals called lignans found in flax seeds oil have anti-inflammatory and antioxidant properties that help reduce the risk of arthritis. Flax seeds are also rich in fiber that helps to ease bowel movement combating constipation and keeping the digestive system healthy.

Use dry roasted and ground flax seeds instead of whole to help your body get the most nutrients from flax seeds for rheumatoid arthritis. This step is necessary to increase their absorption. Whole flax seeds are not easily digestible as their outer shell is hard for the intestines to break down, eating ground flax seeds increase the absorption of the nutrients. Whole flax seeds are chemically stable, but ground flax seeds may go rancid when left exposed to air at room temperature for a longer period, because of oxidation. The best way is to roast and grind them just before the use, to prevent oxidation and increase absorption.

8. Spinach

Vitamin K is a crucial nutrient for joint health. Your body needs vitamin K for healthy bone growth and repair. Lack of vitamin K in the body can increase the risk of osteoarthritis. Spinach is rich in vitamin K, which can help with inflammation caused by arthritis. Spinach is high in bone-preserving calcium. Free radical compounds can destroy healthy cells in the body, and antioxidants destroy those free radicals. Spinach is an excellent source of fiber and antioxidants like vitamins A, C, and E, which protect cells from free radical damage and help reduce inflammation.

Spinach is especially high in the antioxidant kaempferol, an important phytochemical that can bring down the levels of the inflammatory cytokine. Kaempferol inhibits several enzymes that induce oxidative stress that cause rheumatoid arthritis. Study shows kaempferol reduces inflammation and prevents the progression of osteoarthritis. Start adding spinach in your diet to prevent or control arthritis. Avoid eating raw spinach, instead, sauté or blanch them before use. Cooking spinach increases its nutrition value. Also, add 1 tablespoon of lemon juice while blanching. Eating spinach with vitamin C boosts your iron absorption, which exhibits other health benefits.

Read 10 power foods to get rid of anemia in the book "Eat So What! The Power of Vegetarianism."

9. Prebiotic

It is well known that a high-fat diet doubles the body fat percentage and causes obesity. Osteoarthritis in obese people is assumed to be a consequence of undue stress on joints. Researchers have found that obese people have more pro-inflammatory bacteria and almost completely lacked certain beneficial, probiotic bacteria in their guts compared to lean people. This causes inflammation throughout their body, leading to very rapid joint deterioration. These pro-inflammatory bacteria in the gut, which are governed by diet – could be the key driving force behind osteoarthritis. A high-fat diet influences the gut bacteria negatively, allowing harmful bacteria to overgrow. Compared to lean people, osteoarthritis progresses much more quickly in obese people.

Prebiotics are plant fibers. These fibers aren't digestible by humans, so they pass through the digestive system, where they act as fertilizers. They become food for the bacteria and other microbes in the gut and stimulate the growth of healthy bacteria, like Bifidobacteria. The regular consumption of prebiotics foods increases the good bacteria in gut and crowd out bad ones, like pro-inflammatory bacteria. This, in turn, decreases systemic inflammation and slows cartilage breakdown. While prebiotic foods don't reduce obesity, it completely reverses the other symptoms related to arthritis, making the joints more movable. Some examples of prebiotics are banana, apple (don't remove the skin as the skin contains most prebiotic benefits), onion, garlic, oats, asparagus, and yams.

10. Water

Dehydration can make symptoms of arthritis worse. Your joints need fluids to move smoothly. If you are dehydrated, it affects your joints mobility too. Lack of hydration produces friction between the contact point of the joint. Over time, dry cartilage may die and peel from their contact surface of the bones. Drinking more water can improve your arthritis condition for several reasons: water helps to fight inflammation by flushing toxins out of the body. When the joints move, they pull water from the bone marrow to the joint cavity and provides lubrication. If there is not enough water, the joints can't move as they should. Also, water can stimulate the production of synovial fluid that lubricates and cushions the joints and cartilage surrounding them. This keeps the bones from rubbing together, reduces inflammation around the joint, and encourages the growth of new cells in the cartilage tissues. So, increase your water intake to reduce the pain associated with arthritis. For proper lubrication and to control painful symptoms, it is important to drink between two to three liters of water every day, which equals to 8 to 12 glasses of water.

CONCLUSION

Arthritis is no longer a disease of old age. People, even in their late 30s, have started seeing the symptoms of arthritis. The reasons are unhealthy foods that promote inflammation in the body, lack of sunlight exposure, and a diet deficient in anti-inflammatory foods. People who have arthritis can effectively reduce symptoms and inflammation associated with arthritis with the foods mentioned above. These foods can slow down the progression of arthritis and help your body to heal itself. Even if you are a healthy person, you should avoid the inflammation-causing foods and include natural anti-inflammatory foods to prevent arthritis. Anti-inflammatory foods also decrease the risk of autoimmune disorders, diabetes, obesity, cancer, and other diseases.

KEY POINTS

✓ Pain and inflammation are more prominent in the wet season.

✓ Avoid sour food.

✓ Limit your nightshade vegetables.

✓ Eat more omega-3 rich food.

✓ It is important to empty bowel frequently. Constipation aggravates arthritis, pain, and inflammation.

✓ Avoid cold breeze.

✓ Take a hot shower every day. It reduces stiffness by stimulating blood flow to frozen joints and stiff muscles.

✓ Add antioxidant spices to your diet.

UNIT 3

DIET PLAN

Diet Plan for

Healthy and disease-free Life

Diabetes

Hypertension

Arthritis

Diabetes + Hypertension

Hypertension + Arthritis

Diabetes + Arthtitis

DIET PLAN FOR HEALTHY AND DISEASE-FREE LIFE

Diet plan for healthy and disease-free life

- Drink lemon water on an empty stomach.

- Eat overnight soaked dry fruits every day.

  o In winter, 8 almonds + 6 cashews + 6 pistachios + 8 raisins + 2 figs + 4 dates. In summer, (Must be soaked overnight) 5-6 almonds + 4 cashews + 4 pistachios + 4 raisins + 1 fig + 2 dates.

- Drink green tea with lemon juice. If you must add sugar, then add jaggery powder instead of sugar in it.

- Add barley flour to your whole wheat flour in a ratio of 1:7. Add 1 kg barley flour in 7 kg of whole wheat flour.

- Drink more water. Water helps remove toxins from your blood through urine.

- Eat one crushed garlic on an empty stomach once in a week.

- Crush fenugreek seeds and use fenugreek powder in cooking. Fenugreek seeds are bitter in taste, so add 1-2 teaspoon only. If you can tolerate the bitter taste, then add up to 1 tablespoon.

- Use spices such as turmeric, cinnamon, and cumin in cooking.

- Eat one flax seeds laddoo (see in the recipes section) every day.

- Use cold-pressed oil in cooking, such as mustard oil instead of refined oil.

- Use three types of oil- mustard oil for cooking, refined oil such as soybean oil for deep frying, and extra virgin olive oil for sautéing or low flame cooking. Don't use olive oil to deep fry.

- Eat a variety of sprouts.

- Eat seasonal fruits and vegetables, eat them in plenty in season avoid eating non-seasonal fruits and vegetables; they are inferior in nutritional content.

- Drink one glass of milk daily no matter what's your age. Milk is not only required for kids, it is a must for all age groups.

DIET PLAN TO CONTROL DIABETES

Diet plan to control diabetes

- Soak one tablespoon of fenugreek seeds overnight in 250 ml of water. The next morning chew these seeds and drink the fenugreek water. Do this every day (highly effective).

- Chew some (3-4) basil leaves or add them in your morning green tea.

- Eat a handful of overnight soaked nuts.

- Replace potatoes with sweet potatoes and white rice with brown rice.

- Eat one crushed garlic on an empty stomach thrice a week. (after one hour of having soaked fenugreek seeds).

- Add barley flour to your whole wheat flour in a ratio of 1:7. Add 1 kg barley flour in 7 kg of whole wheat flour. Beta-glucan of barley is very effective in preventing diabetes and also prevent weight gain.

- Drink more water, about 2-3 liters, equivalent to 10 -12 glass of 250 ml. Water helps remove excess sugar from your blood through urine, and it helps prevent dehydration.

- In season, drink 50 ml to 100 ml of fresh bitter gourd juice every day. Cook bitter gourd with its peel. Don't remove the skin.

- Eat a variety of sprouts every day.

- Add flax seeds in your dough or add them in yogurt.

- Eat vegetables that have high water content such as bottle gourd and ridge gourd.

- Eat non-starchy vegetables such as carrot, cabbage, cauliflower, green beans, and broccoli.

- Eat vitamin C foods such as amla, lemon, orange, and capsicum.

- Use olive oil, canola oil, and mustard oil in cooking.

- Include apple, oatmeal, and beans in your diet for high soluble fiber.

DIET PLAN TO CONTROL HYPERTENSION

Diet plan to control hypertension

- Add one tablespoon of honey in warm lemon water and drink it on an empty stomach.

- Eat one crushed garlic on an empty stomach every day (if you experience mouth ulcer or heat in the body, reduce the frequency to 5 times a week).

- Soak one tablespoon of fenugreek seeds overnight in 250 ml of water. The next morning chew these seeds and drink the fenugreek water. Do this thrice a week.

- Eat one banana every day, especially if you are taking hypertension medicines.

- Drink green tea and add lemon to it.

- In season, eat multigrain beetroot paratha (see the recipes section). Have 50 to 100 ml of beetroot juice every day.

- Eat a handful of overnight soaked nuts.

- Add barley flour to your whole wheat flour in a ratio of 2:10. Add 200 gm of barley flour to 1 kg of whole wheat flour. Beta-glucan of barley is very effective in preventing hypertension and prevent weight gain.

- In winter, eat plenty of spinach, kale, and chenopodium (bathua).

- Eat one flax seeds laddoo (see in the recipes section) every day.

- Eat plenty of sweet potatoes, especially the purple-fleshed sweet potatoes.

- Eat plenty of legumes such as lentils, chickpeas, kidney beans, and soybeans for potassium, magnesium, and fiber.

- Drink plenty of water, especially on the day you consume more salt.

- Eat fresh fruits, like apples, oranges, and bananas.

- Drink low-fat cow's milk boiled with turmeric powder every night.

- Eat mixed veg raita (see in the recipes section) with lunch.

DIET PLAN TO CONTROL ARTHRITIS

Diet plan to control arthritis

- Take a handful of walnut kernels or two whole walnuts, and two dried figs soaked in water overnight. Eat them on an empty stomach in the morning. Do this every day.

- Eat horse gram (kulthi) as much as possible. Make horse gram dal or powder it and use with your whole wheat flour or add the powder in buttermilk.

- In winter, eat plenty of fresh turmeric roots.

- Drink low-fat cow's milk boiled with turmeric powder at night.

- Eat low-fat plain yogurt.

- Drink green tea mixed with freshly crushed ginger.

- Use canola oil or mustard oil in cooking, avoid sunflower oil and corn oil, which are rich in omega-6 fats.

- Eat sprouted horse gram along with sprouted mung bean, and black chickpeas.

- Eat a handful of soaked nuts, including walnuts, pistachios, almonds, and figs.

- Increase your soybean consumption. Add soybean flour to your whole wheat flour in a ratio of 1:10. Add 1kg of soybean flour to 10 kg of whole wheat flour.

- Eat one flax seeds laddoo (see in the recipes section) every day.

- Eat one crushed garlic on an empty stomach thrice a week.

- Eat plenty of green vegetables including, spinach, kale, and fenugreek leaves.

DIET PLAN TO CONTROL DIABETES + HYPERTENSION

Diet plan to control diabetes + hypertension

- Drink warm lemon water on an empty stomach.

- After half an hour, eat soaked fenugreek seeds and drink the fenugreek water. Do this every day.

- After one hour, eat one crushed garlic. Do this every day.

- Have green tea with added lemon and basil leaves.

- Eat a handful of overnight soaked nuts.

- Drink about 2-3 liters of water in a day.

- Add barley flour to your whole wheat flour in a ratio of 2:10. Add 200 gm of barley flour to 1 kg of whole wheat flour.

- Eat one banana, especially if you are taking hypertension medicines. Don't remove the banana from your diet just because you have diabetes. Cut the sugar intake in tea and other high glycemic fruits.

- In season, drink 50 ml to 100 ml of fresh bitter gourd juice every day.

- In season, eat multigrain beetroot paratha (see the recipes section). Have 50 to 100 ml of beetroot juice every day.

- Eat sprouts every day.

- Add flax seeds in dough or add them in a yogurt fruit salad.

- Eat bottle gourd, carrot, and ridge gourd.

- Replace potatoes with sweet potatoes and eat them in moderation.

- Drink low-fat cow's milk boiled with turmeric powder at night.

- Eat plenty of spinach, kale, cabbage, and chenopodium (bathua).

- Increase legumes consumption, including lentils, chickpeas, kidney beans, and soybeans.

- Eat vitamin C foods such as amla, lemon, orange, and capsicum.

- Use olive oil, canola oil, and mustard oil in cooking.

DIET PLAN TO CONTROL HYPERTENSION + ARTHRITIS

Diet plan to control hypertension + arthritis

- Eat one crushed garlic on an empty stomach every day (if you experience mouth ulcer or heat in the body, reduce the frequency to 5 times a week).

- After half an hour, eat soaked fenugreek seeds and drink the fenugreek water. Do this thrice a week.

- Drink green tea mixed with freshly crushed ginger.

- Eat a handful of overnight soaked dry fruits, including two walnuts, two dried figs, five almonds, four cashew nuts, four pistachios, and four raisins. Eat them daily.

- Drink low-fat turmeric milk at night.

- Eat one banana every day, especially if you are taking hypertension medicines.

- Add barley flour and soybean flour to your whole wheat flour in a ratio 2:1:10. Add 200 gm of barley flour and 100 gm of soybean flour in 1 kg of whole wheat flour.

- Eat plenty of horse gram (kulthi). Make horse gram dal or powder it and use with your whole wheat flour or add the powder in buttermilk.

- In season, eat multigrain beetroot paratha (see the recipes section). Have 50 to 100 ml of beetroot juice every day.

- In winter, eat plenty of fresh turmeric roots, spinach, kale, fenugreek leaves, chenopodium, and sweet potatoes, especially the purple-fleshed sweet potatoes.

- Eat one flax seeds laddoo (see in the recipes section) every day.

- Eat mixed veg raita (see in the recipes section) with lunch.

- Eat plenty of legumes such as lentils, chickpeas, kidney beans, and soybeans for potassium, magnesium, and fiber.

- Drink plenty of water, especially on the day you consume more salt.

- Use extra virgin olive oil (only for shallow fry), canola oil or mustard oil in cooking, avoid sunflower oil and corn oil, which are rich in omega-6 fats.

- Eat fresh fruits, like apples, oranges, and bananas.

DIET PLAN TO CONTROL DIABETES + ARTHRITIS

Diet plan to control diabetes + arthritis

- Soak one tablespoon of fenugreek seeds overnight in 250 ml of water. The next morning chew these seeds and drink the fenugreek water. Do this every day. (highly effective)

- Eat a handful of overnight soaked walnuts and dried figs (2 pieces). Eat them daily.

- Drink green tea mixed with crushed ginger and basil leaves (3-4 leaves).

- Eat one crushed garlic on an empty stomach thrice a week (after one hour of having soaked fenugreek seeds).

- Drink 2-3 liters of water in a day.

- Add barley flour and soybean flour to your whole wheat flour in a ratio of 1.5:1:10. Add 1.5 kg barley flour and 1 kg of soybean flour in 10 kg of whole wheat flour.

- Replace potatoes with sweet potatoes and white rice with brown rice.

- Add horse gram (kulthi) in your diet.

- In winter, eat plenty of fresh turmeric roots. Drink low-fat cow's milk boiled with turmeric powder at night.

- In season, drink 50 ml to 100 ml of fresh bitter gourd juice every day. Cook bitter gourd with its peel. Don't remove the skin.

- Eat sprouted horse gram, sprouted mung bean, and black chickpeas.

- Add flax seeds in dough or add them in the yogurt fruit salad.

- Eat vegetables that have high water content such as bottle gourd and ridge gourd.

- Eat non-starchy vegetables such as carrot, cabbage, cauliflower, green beans, and broccoli.

- Eat plenty of green vegetables including, spinach, kale, and fenugreek leaves.

- Use olive oil, canola oil, and mustard oil in cooking, and avoid sunflower oil and corn oil.

- Include apple, oatmeal, and beans in your diet for high soluble fiber.

UNIT 4

RECIPES

Healthy and tasty recipes to boost your health

BREAKFAST

MULTIGRAIN BEETROOT PARATHA

MIXED VEG RAITA

INSTANT TURMERIC PICKLE

Breakfast

MULTIGRAIN BEETROOT PARATHA

Multigrain beetroot paratha

To make 8 parathas

Ingredients:

Grated beetroot: 1 cup

Grated bottle gourd: 1 cup

Whole wheat flour: 1 cup

Oats flour: 1 cup

Gram flour/chickpea flour: ½ cup

Barley flour: ¼ cup

Amaranth flour: ¼ cup

Salt: To taste

Ginger garlic paste: 1 tablespoon

Jaggery: 2 tablespoons

Coriander powder: 1 teaspoon

Red chili powder: 1 teaspoon

Garam masala: 1 teaspoon

Turmeric: 1 teaspoon

Asafoetida: a pinch

Sesame seeds: 1 tablespoon

Crushed fenugreek seeds: 1 teaspoon

Olive oil: 3 tablespoons

Yogurt: 2 tablespoons (to knead)

Method:

1. Mix all ingredients along with one tablespoon of olive oil in a large mixing bowl.

2. Knead with yogurt and make a stiff dough.

3. Divide the dough into 8 equal balls.

4. Take one piece of the dough ball and dip it in the dry whole wheat flour, dust off the excess flour.

5. Use a rolling pin to roll the dough into a circle.

6. Heat the pan/griddle (tawa) on medium-high flame.

7. Place the paratha on the griddle. Cook for about a minute or cook until the paratha begins puffing up from the base at some places.

8. Flip the paratha and spread 3-4 drops of olive oil. Cook for 2 minutes until it turns light brown.

9. Flip the paratha again and top with 3-4 drops of olive oil, spreading it evenly over the surface. Gently press the paratha with the flat spatula to help the paratha cook evenly.

10. Once you begin to see brown spots on both sides of the paratha, transfer the paratha to a serving plate. Your paratha is ready. Similarly, make all the parathas.

11. Enjoy multigrain beetroot paratha with mixed veg raita.

MIXED VEG RAITA

Mixed veg raita

Ingredients:

Yogurt: 200 grams

Grated beetroot: 1 tablespoon

Finely chopped onion: ¼ cup

Finely chopped tomato: ¼ cup

Finely chopped cabbage: ¼ cup

Finely chopped cucumber: ¼ cup

Brown sugar: 2 tablespoons

Black Salt: 1 teaspoon

Black pepper powder: ½ teaspoon

Red chili powder: ½ teaspoon

Cumin powder: 1 tablespoon

Method:

1. Blend the yogurt and make it smooth.

2. Mix all the veggies except beetroot in yogurt.

3. Add black salt, brown sugar, black pepper powder, red chili powder, and cumin powder in yogurt. Mix well.

4. Keep the raita in the fridge for half an hour.

5. Garnish with grated beetroot.

6. Eat with multigrain beetroot paratha.

INSTANT TURMERIC PICKLE

Instant turmeric pickle

Ingredients:

Fresh turmeric: 100 grams

Lemon juice/Amla juice: 2 tablespoons

Chopped Lemon: 1

Asafoetida: ½ teaspoon

Black Salt: 1 tablespoon

Cumin powder: ½ tablespoon

Black pepper powder: 1 teaspoon

Mustard oil: 2 tablespoons

Method:

1. Wash turmeric to remove any dirt particles. Remove the skin. Chop them finely.

2. Add asafoetida, black salt, cumin powder, black pepper powder, mustard oil, and chopped lemon. Mix well.

3. Add lemon juice or amla juice.

4. Spoon the mixture in a clean and dry glass jar.

5. Cover the jar with a muslin cloth and keep it under sunlight for two days.

6. After two days, turmeric pickle is ready to eat.

7. You can store turmeric pickle in the fridge for up to 1 week.

LUNCH

CHOLE MASALA

NON-FRIED OATS BHATURE

FLAX SEEDS LADDOO

Lunch

CHOLE MASALA

Chole masala

Serves 4

Ingredients:

To cook chickpeas

Uncooked dried Chickpeas: 200 grams

Teabags: 3

Onion: 1 medium

Salt: To taste

Water: 500 ml

For gravy

Garlic: 12 cloves

Ginger: 2 inches

Onion: 3 medium size

Asafoetida: ½ teaspoon

Cumin: 1 teaspoon

Bay leaves – 1

Coriander Powder- 1 teaspoon

Turmeric powder: 1 teaspoon

Red chili powder: 1 teaspoon

Garam Masala- 1 teaspoon

Chole Masala- 2 tablespoons

Dry mango powder: 1 teaspoon

Brown sugar: 1 tablespoon (optional)

Salt: To taste

Water: 300 ml

Mustard oil: 2 tablespoons

Method:

1. Soak the chickpeas in enough water. Keep it overnight or for at least 8 hours.

2. Next morning, drain the water and rinse chickpeas thoroughly.

3. In a pressure cooker, add the soaked chickpeas, tea bags, salt, sliced onion (1 medium), and 500 ml water. Pressure cook at medium flame for 5-6 whistles. It will take around 15 minutes. The chickpeas should be soft when you mash it with a spoon.

4. If chickpeas are hard, pressure cook them for two whistles.

5. Strain the chickpeas and keep the stock for later use.

6. Grind onion, garlic, ginger, together to make a smooth paste.

7. Add mustard oil to the hot pan, add asafoetida, cumin, and bay leaves. Sauté for 2-3 minutes.

8. Add the onion mixture in the oil. Mix well and cover the pan with a lid. Cook at the medium-low flame for 15 minutes. Cook till it leaves oil. The raw taste of onion should evaporate completely.

9. Add turmeric powder, coriander powder, dry mango powder, red chili powder, sugar, salt (keep in mind, we have added salt while cooking chickpeas too), garam masala, and chole masala (skip it if you don't have chole masala). Add another teaspoon of garam masala if you are not adding chole masala.

10. Cook for 2-3 minutes.

11. Add chickpeas, mix well. Masala mixture should coat the chickpeas entirely.

12. Cover it and cook for 5-7 minutes.

13. Add the stock in which chickpeas were cooked. Add another 300 ml of water. Water should be just above the chickpeas. Don't add too much water, it will dilute the taste.

14. Take a masher and mash almost 20% of chickpeas to make the gravy thick.

15. Cover it and cook for 18-20 minutes on low flame until chickpeas absorb the flavor of masala. The gravy should be thick.

16. Your chole masala is ready to eat. Eat it with non-fried oats bhature or brown rice.

NON-FRIED OATS BHATURE

Non-fried oats bhature

Serves 4

Ingredients:

Oats: 2 ½ cup

Whole wheat flour: 1 ½ cup

Salt: To taste

Brown sugar: 1 teaspoon

Baking powder: 1 teaspoon

Baking soda: 1 teaspoon

Thick yogurt: 1 cup

Olive oil – 1 tablespoon + for making bhature

Method:

1. Grind the oats. Mix with whole wheat flour in a large bowl. Add salt, sugar, baking powder, baking soda, and oil. Mix well.

2. Add 1 cup of thick yogurt and knead for 5-6 minutes. The dough should be a little stiff for making crispy bhature. If required, add more yogurt.

3. Cover the dough with a wet muslin cloth. Leave it for at least 2 hours.

4. Divide the dough into 15 equal parts.

5. Grease your palm well with oil. Take 1 part and make a ball shape between your palm. Smoothen the ball, make sure it's crack free.

6. Repeat the process for all parts.

7. Now take 1 ball and roll it into oval shape or round discs. It should neither be too thick nor thin.

8. Heat a griddle. Grease it with oil. Put bhatura on a hot greased griddle.

9. First, cook one side. Turn the bhatura and add 1 teaspoon of oil to make it crisp from the other side too. Cook the other side. Brown spots should appear on both sides.

10. Repeat with the remaining dough to make 14 more bhature.

11. Eat non-fried oats bhature with chole masala.

FLAX SEEDS LADDOO

Flax seeds laddoo

To make 25 laddoos

Ingredients:

Flax seeds: 500 grams

Tragacanth gum/gond: 100 grams (optional)

Chopped Almonds: 100 grams

Chopped Walnuts: 100 grams

Jaggery: 250 grams

Cow's Ghee/Clarified butter: 4 tablespoons

Method:

1. Dry roast flax seeds on low flame until it slightly changes its color and releases the roasted aroma.

2. Allow the roasted flax seeds to cool down and grind in a mixer.

3. Grate the jaggery and keep aside.

4. Heat ghee in a pan. Fry gond in the ghee till it swells.

5. Remove gond from ghee. Cool it down and break it in mortar pestle or with your hand.

6. In the remaining ghee, add chopped almonds and walnuts. Fry till they turn slightly brown.

7. Remove the nuts and add grated jaggery in the same remaining ghee.

8. Cook for 3-5 minutes till jaggery dissolves. Once jaggery gets dissolved, switch off the flame immediately. Don't cook jaggery after it dissolves; otherwise, your laddoos will be too hard to eat.

9. Now add the ground flax seeds, almonds, walnuts, and gond to it. Mix well.

10. Make round shape laddoo with hands while the mixture is hot.

11. If your laddoos are not binding well, then heat the mixture for 2 minutes.

12. Enjoy your flax seeds laddoos. Store the remaining laddoos under refrigeration and consume within two weeks.

NOTE FROM LA FONCEUR

Dear Reader,

Thank you for reading *Eat to Prevent and Control Disease*. I hope you have found this book helpful.

If you liked the book, please leave a review online. Help other health-conscious readers find this book by telling them why you enjoyed reading. Your help in spreading awareness will be gratefully received.

Join my mailing list at www.eatsowhat.com/mailing-list

If you are looking for a permanent solution to your hair problems, read *Secret of Healthy Hair*.

Learn how a vegetarian diet can be the solution to a disease-free healthy life in Eat So What! series- *Eat So What! The Power of Vegetarianism* and *Eat So What! Smart Ways to Stay Healthy*.

All of my books are available in eBook, paperback, and hardcover editions.

Regards

La Fonceur

REFERENCES

1. Soheil Z, Habsah A, "A Review on Antibacterial, Antiviral, and Antifungal Activity of Curcumin." Biomed Res Int. 2014; 2014: 186864.
2. Silagy C, Neil A, "Garlic as a lipid lowering agent--a meta-analysis." R Coll Physicians Lond. Jan-Feb 1994;28(1):39-45.
3. Matthias B, Mandy S, "Fiber and magnesium intake and incidence of type 2 diabetes: a prospective study and meta-analysis." Arch Intern Med. 2007 May 14;167(9):956-65.
4. Karin R, Toben C, Fakler P, "Effect of garlic on serum lipids: an updated meta-analysis." Nutr Rev. 2013 May;71(5):282-99.
5. Holly L, Sharon A, "Garlic and onions: Their cancer prevention properties." Cancer Prev Res (Phila). 2015 Mar; 8(3): 181-189.
6. Ranade M, Mudgalkar N, "A simple dietary addition of fenugreek seed leads to the reduction in blood glucose levels: A parallel-group, randomized single-blind trial." Ayu. 2017 Jan-Jun; 38(1-2): 24-27.
7. Calado A, Neves M, "The Effect of Flaxseed in Breast Cancer: A Literature Review." Front Nutr. 2018; 5: 4.
8. Chikako M, Taeko K, "Effects of glycolipids from spinach on mammalian DNA polymerases." Biochem Pharmacol. 2003 Jan 15;65(2):259-67.
9. Mondal S, Varma S, "Double-blinded randomized controlled trial for immunomodulatory effects of Tulsi (Ocimum sanctum Linn.) leaf extract on healthy volunteers." Ethnopharmacol. 2011 Jul 14;136(3):452-
10. Dokania M, Kishore K, Sharma PK, "Effect of Ocimum sanctum extract on sodium nitrite-induced experimental amnesia in mice." Thai J Pharma Sci. 2011; 35:123-30.
11. Eddouks M, Amina B, "Antidiabetic plants improving insulin sensitivity." J Pharm Pharmacol. 2014 Sep;66(9):1197-214.
12. Widjaja S, Rusdiana, "Glucose Lowering Effect of Basil Leaves in Diabetic Rats." J Med Sci. 2019 May 15; 7(9): 1415-1417.
13. A review on, "What You Need to Know about Dietary Supplements." https://www.fda.gov/food/
14. Gallagher J, Vinod Yalamanchili V, "The Effect of Vitamin D on Calcium Absorption in Older Women." J Clin Endocrinol Metab. 2012 Oct; 97(10): 3550-3556.
15. Gupta R, Gangoliya S, "Reduction of phytic acid and enhancement of bioavailable micronutrients in food grains." J Food Sci Technol. 2015 Feb; 52(2): 676-684.
16. Lee A, Thurnham D, "Consumption of tomato products with olive oil but not sunflower oil increases the antioxidant activity of plasma." Free Radical Biol Med. 2000 Nov 15;29(10):1051-5.

17. Malouf M, Grimley E, "Folic acid with or without vitamin B12 for cognition and dementia." Cochrane Database Syst Rev, 2003;(4): CD004514.

18. Abularrage C, Sidawy A, "Effect of folic Acid and vitamins B6 and B12 on microcirculatory vasoreactivity in patients with hyperhomocysteinemia." Vasc Endovascular Surg. 2007 Aug-Sep;41(4):339-45.

19. Sarwar N, Gao P, "Diabetes mellitus, fasting blood glucose concentration, and risk of vascular disease: a collaborative meta-analysis of 102 prospective studies. Emerging Risk Factors Collaboration." Lancet. 2010; 26; 375:2215-2222.

20. Bourne R, Stevens G, "Causes of vision loss worldwide, 1990-2010: a systematic analysis." Lancet Global Health 2013;1:e339-e349

21. "Diabetes facts & figures." The International Diabetes Federation (IDF), 2020, https://www.idf.org/aboutdiabetes/what-is-diabetes/facts-figures.html

22. Cruz K, Oliveira A, "Antioxidant role of zinc in diabetes mellitus." World J Diabetes. 2015 Mar 15; 6(2): 333-337.

23. Abdelsalam S, Hesham M, "The Role of Protein Tyrosine Phosphatase (PTP)-1B in Cardiovascular Disease and Its Interplay with Insulin Resistance." Biomolecules. 2019 Jul; 9(7): 286.

24. Alam MD, Uddin R, "Beneficial Role of Bitter Melon Supplementation in Obesity and Related Complications in Metabolic Syndrome." J Lipids. 2015; 2015: 496169.

25. Padmaja Chaturvedi P, "Antidiabetic potentials of Momordica charantia: multiple mechanisms behind the effects." J Med Food. 2012 Feb;15(2):101-7.

26. Joseph B, Jini D, "Antidiabetic effects of Momordica charantia (bitter melon) and its medicinal potency." Asian Pac J Trop Dis. 2013 Apr; 3(2): 93-102.

27. Tayyab F, Lal S, "Medicinal plants and its impact on diabetes." World J Pharm Res. 2012;1(4):1019-1046.

28. Paul A, Raychaudhuri S, "Medicinal uses and molecular identification of two Momordica charantia varieties - a review." E J Bio. 2010;6(2):43-51.

29. Garg A, "High-monounsaturated-fat diets for patients with diabetes mellitus: a meta-analysis." Am J Clin Nutr, 1998 Mar;67(3 Suppl):577S-582S.

30. Kassaian N, Azadbakht L, "Effect of fenugreek seeds on blood glucose and lipid profiles in type 2 diabetic patients." Int J Vitam Nutr Res. 2009 Jan;79(1):34-9.

31. Kesika P, Sivamaruthi B, "Do Probiotics Improve the Health Status of Individuals with Diabetes Mellitus? A Review on Outcomes of Clinical Trials." Biomed Res Int. 2019; 2019: 1531567.

32. D'souza J, D'souza P, "Anti-diabetic effects of the Indian indigenous fruit Emblica Officinalis Gaertn: active constituents and modes of action." Food Funct. 2014 Apr;5(4):635-44.

33. Sharabi K, Tavares C, "Molecular Pathophysiology of Hepatic Glucose Production," Mol Aspects Med. 2015 Dec; 46: 21-33.

34. Santhi K, Rajamani S, "Amla, a Marvelous Fruit for Type -2 Diabetics-A Review." Int. J. Curr. Microbiol. App. Sci. 2017, 5:116-123

35. Radzeviciene L, Ostrauskas R, "Adding Salt to Meals as a Risk Factor of Type 2 Diabetes Mellitus: A Case-Control Study." Nutrients. 2017 Jan; 9(1): 67.

36. Li J, Zhang N, "Non-steroidal anti-inflammatory drugs increase insulin release from beta cells by inhibiting ATP-sensitive potassium channels." Br J Pharmacol. 2007 Jun; 151(4): 483-493.

37. Kato Y, Domoto T, "Effect on Blood Pressure of Daily Lemon Ingestion and Walking." J Nutr Metab. 2014; 2014: 912684.

38. Dehkordi F, Kamkhah A, "Antihypertensive effect of Nigella sativa seed extract in patients with mild hypertension." Fundam Clin Pharmacol, 2008 Aug;22(4):447-52.

39. Diego A, Ocampo B, "Dietary Nitrate from Beetroot Juice for Hypertension: A Systematic Review." Biomolecules. 2018 Dec; 8(4): 134.

40. Ried K, Fakler P, "Potential of garlic (Allium sativum) in lowering high blood pressure: mechanisms of action and clinical relevance." Integr Blood Press Control. 2014; 7: 71-82.

41. Aluko E, Olubobokun T, "Honey's Ability to Reduce Blood Pressure and Heart Rate in Healthy Male Subjects." Frontiers in Science, 2014

42. Jovanovski E, Bosco L, "Effect of Spinach, a High Dietary Nitrate Source, on Arterial Stiffness and Related Hemodynamic Measures: A Randomized, Controlled Trial in Healthy Adults." Clin Nutr Res. 2015 Jul; 4(3): 160-167.

43. Hekmatpou D, Mortaji S, "The Effectiveness of Olive Oil in Controlling Morning Inflammatory Pain of Phalanges and Knees Among Women with Rheumatoid Arthritis: A Randomized Clinical Trial." Rehabil Nurs. Mar/Apr 2020;45(2):106-113.

44. Rajagopal V, Pushpan C, "Comparative effect of horse gram and black gram on inflammatory mediators and antioxidant," Journal of Food and Drug Analysis, 2017, Pages 845-853

45. Huang Q, Mao-Jie Wang M, "Can active components of licorice, glycyrrhizin and glycyrrhetinic acid, lick rheumatoid arthritis." Oncotarget, 2016 Jan 12; 7(2): 1193-1202.

IMPORTANT TERMINOLOGY

Arteries: Arteries are blood vessels that carry oxygen-rich blood from the heart to the body.

Vascular: Vascular is related to vessels that carry blood in the body.

Vasoconstriction: Vaso means vessels, so vasoconstriction means narrowing of the blood vessels.

Vasodilation: Dilation or widening of blood vessels.

Glucose: Glucose means sweet in Greek. It is a type of sugar. You get carbohydrates from foods, which break down into glucose, and your body uses it for energy.

Hyperglycemia: Hyperglycemia refers to high levels of sugar (glucose) in the blood.

Bioavailability: The actual proportion of a substance that reaches the blood circulation after it introduced into the body to show its effect.

Free radicals: Free radicals are the unpaired electrons that form due to the oxidative process in the body. These unpaired electrons like to be in pairs, so they pair with the electrons in proteins and DNA and damage them.

Antioxidants: Body has antioxidants, which neutralize free radicals by inhibiting the oxidative process that forms free radicals.

Oxidative stress: When free radicals outnumber the naturally occurring antioxidants, it results in oxidative stress. This imbalance leads to cell and tissue damage, including DNA, protein, and lipids. Damage to your DNA increases your risk of chronic diseases such as cancer, rheumatoid arthritis, diabetics, stroke, and aging.

Inflammation: Inflammation is the response of the body to harmful pathogens, and irritants, and eliminate the initial cause of cell injury. Body releases white blood cells to heal the damaged cells. When the immune system mistakenly attacks healthy tissue, it causes harmful abnormal inflammation. Reasons for abnormal inflammation are stress, smoking, and alcohol consumption. Some examples of diseases associated with abnormal inflammations are rheumatoid arthritis, psoriasis, and inflammatory bowel diseases.

ABBREVIATIONS

RA- Rheumatoid Arthritis

BP- Blood pressure

LDL- Low-density lipoproteins

HDL- High-density lipoprotein

COX- Cyclooxygenase

PG- Prostaglandin

RAAS- Renin–angiotensin–aldosterone system

ABOUT THE AUTHOR

La Fonceur is the author of the book series *Eat So What!* and *Secret of Healthy* **Hair**, a dance artist, and a health blogger. She has a master's degree in Pharmacy. She specialized in Pharmaceutical Technology and worked as a research scientist in the research and development department. She has published an article titled 'Techniques for Producing Biotechnology-Derived Products of Pharmaceutical Use' in Pharmtechmedica Journal. She is also a registered pharmacist. Being a research scientist, she has worked closely with drugs. Based on her experience, she believes that one can prevent most of the diseases with nutritious vegetarian foods and a healthy lifestyle.

ALL BOOKS BY LA FONCEUR

Full-length books:

Mini editions:

Hindi editions:

CONNECT WITH LA FONCEUR

Instagram: **@la_fonceur** | **@eatsowhat**

Facebook: **LaFonceur** | **eatsowhat**

Twitter: **@la_fonceur**

Amazon Author Page:

www.amazon.com/La-Fonceur/e/B07PM8SBSG/

Bookbub Author Page:
www.bookbub.com/authors/la-fonceur

Sign up to my website to get exclusive offers on my books:

Blog: **www.eatsowhat.com**

Website: **www.lafonceur.com/sign-up**

www.ingramcontent.com/pod-product-compliance
Lightning Source LLC
Chambersburg PA
CBHW030823270326
41928CB00007B/863